CON
HYPERTENSION

An Illustrated Guide to Understanding
Treatment and Control of High Blood Pressure

R. BRIAN HAYNES, MD, PhD
FRANS H. H. LEENEN, MD, PhD

1994
Empowering Press, Hamilton, Canada

Canadian Cataloguing in Publication Data

Haynes, R. Brian (Robert Brian), 1947 –
Conquering Hypertension: an illustrated guide to understanding treatment
and control of high blood pressure

Includes Index.
ISBN 0-9697781-2-0

1. Hypertension - Treatment.   I. Leenen, Frans H. H.   II. Title.
R685.H8H38 1994   616.1'3206   C94-932614-3

Published by:
Empowering Press
Hamilton, Ontario, Canada

The opinions expressed in this book are those of the authors. Readers are
advised to consult with a physician prior to acting on the basis of material
contained herein. The authors and Empowering Press hereby disclaim responsibility for any loss suffered by any person as a result of failing to consult with
a physician.

Astra Pharma Inc. edition published under the title *Down with High Blood
Pressure.*

Printed in Canada

CONTENTS

Darlene Abbott, RN, MSc, is a nurse-specialist at Foothills Hospital, Calgary, and is currently vice-president of the Canadian Coalition for High Blood Pressure Prevention and Control.

Martin J. Bass, MD, MSc, FCFP, is director of the Centre for Studies in Family Medicine at the University of Western Ontario, London, Canada. He is a professor of family medicine and of epidemiology who practices at the Byron Family Medical Centre in London. He is a former board member of the Canadian Hypertension Society. His research interests include home blood pressure monitoring and non-drug approaches to blood pressure control.

Jean-Hughes Brossard, MD, FRCPC, is a research fellow at McGill University and staff endocrinologist at St. Luc Hospital in Montreal, Quebec.

S. George Carruthers, MD, FRCPC, is chair of the Department of Medicine at Dalhousie University. Dr. Carruthers is a past-president of the Canadian Hypertension Society and sees patients at the Victoria General Hospital.

Arun Chockalingham, MS, PhD, is a research consultant with Health Canada, Preventive Health.

A. Mark Clarfield, MD, CCFP, FRCPC, is currently director of academic affairs at Sarah Herzog Memorial Hospital and head of geriatrics (Ministry of Health) in Jerusalem. Previously he was head of geriatrics at McGill University, Montreal, Quebec.

Jean Cléroux, PhD, FACSM, is assistant professor of medicine, Faculty of Medicine, Université Laval, and senior researcher, Hypertension Research Unit, Centre Hospitalier de l'Université Laval Research Centre, Ville de Québec, Québec.

C.R. (Tim) Dean, MD, DPhil, FRCPC, is associate professor of medicine at Dalhousie University and director of the Hypertension Unit, Camp Hill Medical Centre in Halifax, Nova Scotia.

C. Edward Evans, MB, MRCS, FCFP, is a professor of family medicine at McMaster University. He has written a summary for practicing physicians of the Canadian Hypertension Society's Consensus Conference Recommendations and has done research on home blood pressure devices.

J. George Fodor, MD, PhD, FRCPC, is a cardiologist and clinical epidemiologist who was seeing patients in the Hypertension Clinic of the St. John's (Newfoundland) General Hospital. At present, he is a consultant (research) at the Ottawa Heart Institute. He is a past-president of the Canadian Hypertension Society.

Pavel Hamet, MD, PhD, FRCPC, is professor of medicine, physiology and nutrition at the Université de Montréal and director of the Research Centre of Hôtel-Dieu de Montréal. He is a past-president of the Canadian Hypertension Society and current secretary of the International Society of Hypertension.

R. Brian Haynes, MD, PhD, FRCPC, is professor of clinical epidemiology and medicine at McMaster University and sees patients with high blood pressure at Chedoke-McMaster Hospital in Hamilton, Ontario. He is a past-president of the Canadian Hypertension Society.

Jane Irvine, DPhil, CPsych, is a psychologist at The Toronto Hospital and an assistant professor of psychiatry, Faculty of Medicine, University of Toronto. In her clinical practice she sees patients with high blood pressure and/or cardio-vascular disease.

Pierre Larochelle, MD, PhD, FRCPC, is professor of pharmacology at the Université de Montréal and director of a hypertension clinic at the Hotel-Dieu de Montréal. He is the president of the Québec Hypertension Society and president-elect of the Canadian Hypertension Society.

Frans H.H. Leenen, MD, PhD, FRCPC, is professor of medicine and pharma-cology at the University of Ottawa, and sees patients with high blood pressure at the University of Ottawa Heart Institute. He is a past-president of the Canadian Hypertension Society.

Mitchell A.H. Levine, MD, MSc, FRCPC, is associate professor of clinical epi-demiology and medicine at McMaster University and sees patients with high blood pressure at St. Joseph's Hospital in Hamilton, Ontario.

Alexander G. Logan, MD, FRCPC, is professor of medicine at the University of Toronto, head of clinical epidemiology in the Samuel Lunenfeld Research Institute, and sees patients with high blood pressure at Mount Sinai Hospital in Toronto, Ontario. He is a past-president of the Canadian Hypertension Society.

Martin G. Myers, MD, FRCPC, is a professor of medicine at the University of Toronto and a cardiologist at Sunnybrook Health Science Centre in Toronto. He is a past-president of the Canadian Hypertension Society.

Jack Onrot, MD, FRCPC, is a clinical pharmacologist at St. Paul's Hospital in Vancouver, BC. He practices internal medicine and has a special interest in patients with blood pressure problems.

Richard A. Reeves, MD, FRCPC, saw patients at Sunnybrook Hospital, University of Toronto, where he was assistant professor of medicine and pharmacology until he moved to the Bristol-Myers Squibb Pharmaceutical Research Institute, Princeton, New Jersey, in 1993 as director of Cardiovascular Clinical Research, Hypertension/Renal Division.

Louise F. Roy, MD, FRCPC, is assistant professor of medicine at the Université de Montréal and sees patients with renal diseases and high blood pressure at St. Luc's Hospital in Montréal, Québec.

Douglas R. Ryan, MD, FRCPC, is assistant professor of medicine at the University of Toronto and associate staff physician at the Mount Sinai Hospital Hypertension Clinic in Toronto, Ontario.

David L. Sackett, MD, FRSC, FRCPC, after several years at McMaster University in Canada, is now professor of clinical epidemiology in the Nuffield Department of Medicine at the University of Oxford in England, where he practices medicine, teaches, and continues his research into diagnosis and therapy.

Beverley Whitmore, RD, is a registered dietitian and works in the Hypertension Clinic at the Foothills Hospital in Calgary.

Tom Wilson, MD, FRCPC, is a professor of pharmacology and medicine at the University of Saskatchewan. He practices internal medicine and is director of the Cardiovascular Risk Factor Reduction Unit.

R. Brian Haynes, MD, PhD,

and Frans H.H. Leenen, MD, PhD

On behalf of the Canadian Hypertension Society (CHS), we are proud to present a book for people who have high blood pressure (hypertension★) or who want to know about this common problem. This is the third book we have published since 1986 as part of the public education program of the Society and reflects the rapid pace of important advances in knowledge about the management of high blood pressure. The current book was prompted by a major CHS conference on high blood pressure at which experts reviewed all previous recommendations for high blood pressure in the light of new evidence from clinical research among people with high blood pressure. Many of the previous recommendations had to be modified because of the new evidence. This book summarizes all of the recommendations, including the new ones. The most important advances have come in our understanding of the management of hypertension in the elderly and among diabetics, and in the importance of dealing with related risks to cardiovascular health including smoking, high cholesterol, and obesity. The recommendations from the experts convened to address these topics are explained in the chapters of this book.

The response from people with high blood pressure and the public to our previous books was very positive. It convinced us that people with high blood pressure do want detailed information about their condition. We also hope that the information in this book will put patients and their doctors on the "same wavelength". The CHS also has prepared

---

★ The terms "high blood pressure" and "hypertension" mean the same thing: a sustained increase in blood pressure. Hypertension does *not* mean that a person is "hyper" or "tense", and high blood pressure is seldom caused by "stress" or anxiety.

articles, information kits and a videotape for doctors so that they will have information based on the same, strong evidence on which this book is based.

Hypertension from the Perspective of Today's Patients

Of all the many advances in health care over the last three decades, none is more remarkable than the development of effective treatments for high blood pressure. Before these treatments became available, people who had high blood pressure were at high risk of strokes, heart failure, heart attacks, and kidney failure, causing both suffering and premature loss of life. Now, *with good care*, many of these complications can be avoided.

Unfortunately, the treatments for high blood pressure are still not perfect. First, they do not cure the condition. Rather, they bring the blood pressure down to normal levels, but only while they are being taken regularly. Some people find taking medical treatments on a daily basis an unbearable nuisance. Second, the medications can cause adverse effects. Some patients refuse to take pills entirely, and try to get by with non-drug treatments such as weight reduction, low salt diets, giving up alcohol and "taking it easy". Alas, these treatments often are less effective than medications — and are often much more of a nuisance. They can, nonetheless, often complement drug treatments and reduce the need for medication.

Fortunately, there are many treatment options for high blood pressure. By matching the treatments to the individual's characteristics and responses, it is usually possible to find a successful match: good blood pressure control with few or no adverse effects.

Achieving the best match takes teamwork. If you have

high blood pressure, the members of the team are you and your doctor, and often members of your family. Nurses, pharmacists and dietitians may also become members of your team. Your doctor's job is to know about high blood pressure, its causes and management, and to know enough about you to prescribe the treatment or treatments that best fit your circumstances. Your tasks are to know enough about high blood pressure to help in this process, to follow the treatment as prescribed (or tell your doctor if you are unable to follow it), and to report any adverse effects that you feel the treatment may be causing. Your doctor may give you additional tasks such as measuring your own blood pressure.

This book provides the facts you will need to understand the nature of high blood pressure, its (potential) complications, and the details of its diagnosis, treatments and monitoring. This information will help you to keep up your end of the teamwork (or "therapeutic alliance") that is needed to keep your blood pressure under control with a minimum of side-effects and a minimum of fuss.

About the Authors

The authors of the book are all members of the Canadian Hypertension Society, an organization dedicated to research and education in hypertension and optimal care of people with high blood pressure. Our names and affiliations appear in the front matter of the book. Most of us are health professionals — physicians, nurses, dietitians. Most are also involved in research, attempting to generate new knowledge about high blood pressure. All of us teach students in the health sciences about hypertension. Finally, we all try to teach our patients about high blood pressure — that is why we have written this book.

About the Book

The book provides an overview of high blood pressure for the public in general and people with high blood pressure in particular. While some readers may want to read the whole book, others may want to read only the chapters of special interest to them. For those who want to select specific chapters, the following guide may help.

The first chapter describes the nature of high blood pressure and its effects on the body. If you don't know anything about why the body needs blood pressure or what high blood pressure is, this is the place to start. However, the chapter does not have much practical information about what you can do to help with the treatment of your high blood pressure.

The second chapter provides a practical guide on how blood pressure is measured and how hypertension is diagnosed. It then explains the questions doctors ask and tests they order when they see someone with newly discovered hypertension.

Chapter 3 summarizes the evidence that treatment for high blood pressure does more good than harm. If you have any doubts that blood pressure-lowering treatments are beneficial to your health and longevity, be sure to read this chapter. We think you will be convinced!

Chapter 4 is about diet and hypertension. Diet is an aspect of lifestyle, of course. But it is so important to our health that we have given it its own chapter.

Chapter 5 summarizes the relationship between "lifestyle" (stress, exercise, smoking, alcohol) and high blood pressure. It then provides a practical guide on how you can modify your lifestyle to lower your blood pressure.

Chapter 6 describes the current Canadian Hypertension Society recommendations for medications for high blood pressure. It is a summary of the same information given to physicians.

Chapters 7 to 11 provide specific details about the many medications that are prescribed to lower blood pressure. Here you will find out about the effectiveness of the medications and their individual advantages and disadvantages, including their side-effects.

Chapters 12 to 14 provide special information for specific groups. Chapter 12 is for the elderly, Chapter 13 for diabetics and Chapter 14 for women who are pregnant or on birth control pills.

Finally, Chapter 15 gives practical tips on what you can do to benefit most from treatment for your hypertension. This chapter is a "must" for everyone receiving therapy for high blood pressure.

About the Sponsor for the Book

This book has been prepared with the assistance of an educational grant from Astra Pharma Incorporated, a pharmaceutical company that makes many drugs, including some that are useful for the treatment of hypertension. We are grateful for Astra's aid, which was of particular help in publicizing the book and making it available to physicians for their patients.

We are also grateful for Astra's agreement to, and insistence on, the writing arrangements for the book. The material in the book is entirely the responsibility of the authors, on behalf of the Canadian Hypertension Society. A concerted attempt has been made to represent all aspects of hypertension impartially, according to scientific merit, including all drug and non-drug treatments.

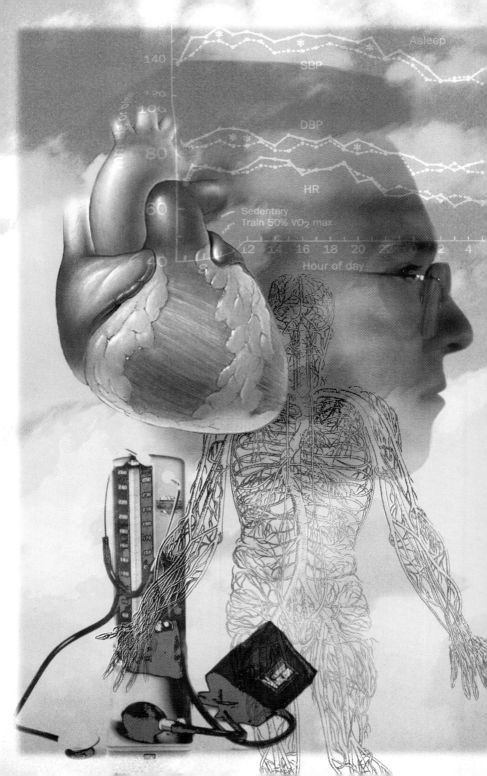

Asleep

SBP

DBP

HR

Sedentary
Train 50% VO₂ max

140

120

100

80

60

40

12 14 16 18 20   2   4

Hour of day

CHAPTER 1

HIGH BLOOD PRESSURE AND THE HUMAN BODY

Mitchell A. H. Levine, MD, MSc, and
J. George Fodor, MD, PhD

As the term indicates, blood pressure is the pressure by which the blood is circulated in blood vessels. The heart is a muscular pump that supplies the pressure to move the blood along. Blood vessels have elastic walls and provide some resistance to the flow. Hence, there is pressure in the system even between heart beats.

"Nature's purpose" in keeping blood pressure at a certain level is to ensure that the blood, which carries nutrients and oxygen, is pumped to various organs. Blood pressure is highest in the larger arteries and lower in the smaller blood vessels. It also varies throughout the day, increasing during exercise, mental stress and sexual intercourse, and decreasing when the body is resting during sleep.

The first measurements of blood pressure in human blood vessels were taken by inserting a tube into an artery, an inconvenient, somewhat dangerous, and painful method. General use of blood pressure readings was made possible by the development of so-called "indirect techniques", particularly an inflatable cuff like the tube in a tire. The blood pressure is determined by inflating the cuff around a limb, usually the upper arm. One end of a listening device such as a stethoscope is placed over an artery "downstream" to the cuff, and the other end of the *stethoscope* is placed in the ears of the observer. When the cuff pressure is greater than the blood pressure in the limb, the blood cannot flow past the cuff and no pulse sounds can be heard. When the cuff pressure is just below that pressure level the blood can flow past the cuff again and pulse sounds can be heard through the stethoscope.

The pressure at which the first pulse sound can be heard

is called *systolic* blood pressure. As the pressure in the cuff is decreased, the pulse sounds continue to be heard for awhile and then they disappear again. The pressure level when the sounds disappear is the *diastolic* pressure. Blood pressure usually is indicated as two numbers, for example, 130/80. The first number is the systolic and the second number is the diastolic blood pressure, expressed in millimetres of mercury (mm Hg). There is more information on measuring blood pressure in Chapter 2 and instructions on how you can measure your own blood pressure in Chapter 15.

How Is Blood Pressure Kept Normal?

The mechanisms by which blood pressure is maintained are complicated, and it is not surprising that they are not fully understood. If you would like to know about them, read on. Otherwise you might want to skip to the next section, High Blood Pressure.

Blood pressure is controlled mainly by the brain, the autonomic nervous system, the kidneys, some of the endocrine glands, the arteries, and the heart (Fig. 1-1). The *brain* is the centre of blood pressure control in the body. It directs the various other organs in response to the body's demands and needs. Nerve fibres that are part of the *autonomic nervous system* bring signals from all parts of the body to inform the brain of the status of the blood pressure, the volume of blood and the specialized needs of all organs. This information is processed by the brain and decisions are automatically taken and messages sent out via the outgoing nerves. These nerves departing from the brain end up in the organs, including the blood vessels, where the signals cause narrowing or opening of the vessels. These nerves function automatically, without our knowledge, unlike other nerves that we can control, such as those needed for physical movements of the body. The blood pressure can be affected at many levels in the brain centre, on the way to and from the autonomic nervous system or during the process of sending messages to the blood vessels.

The *kidney* is the regulator of fluids in the body. This organ has many special duties and is designed to help us survive as creatures who live out of the sea, as it can keep the necessary amount of salt and water in the body while getting rid of excess fluids as well as body wastes.

The kidney makes a hormone called *renin* that causes the blood pressure to rise in response to anything that lowers the

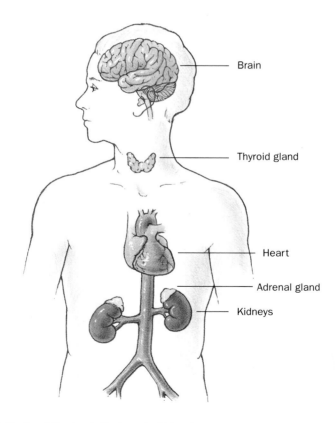

Brain

Thyroid gland

Heart

Adrenal gland

Kidneys

Figure 1-1: Parts of the body that control blood pressure

blood pressure and thereby threatens the normal function of the kidney. Renin from the kidney stimulates the formation of *angiotensin*. Angiotensin causes blood vessels to constrict and in turn the blood pressure rises. *Hormones* from several organs also affect the blood pressure. On top of the kidneys sits a small gland called the *adrenal* gland. It secretes several hormones that can raise blood pressure, including *cortisone*, *adrenaline* and *aldosterone*. The thyroid gland produces *thyroid* hormone or *thyroxine*, which is also important in blood pressure control. The ovaries secrete *estrogen*, which tends to raise blood pressure (see Chapter 14). Although the heart's main function is to pump blood to the body's organs, it also functions as an endocrine gland. It secretes *natriuretic* hormone, a substance that can rid the body of excess salt and help keep the blood vessels properly dilated. All of these hormones are necessary for the body to function. It is only when they are excreted in abnormal amounts that they cause the blood pressure to become inappropriately elevated.

The *arteries* themselves also contribute to blood pressure control. These are elastic tubes that distribute the blood throughout the body to the organs. The muscles in the walls of the vessels can dilate to increase the blood supply to an organ, or contract to shunt blood away and distribute it where it is most needed. For example, when we eat, blood is shifted to the bowel to help with digestion. When we exercise, it is shifted to the exercising muscles, while at the same time maintaining an adequate amount of blood for the brain and other vital organs.

The functions of the kidney, hormones and arteries are not isolated. As mentioned already, they are directed by the brain. However, they also use their own systems to inform each other of their needs. For example, the kidney's secretion of renin is influenced by the brain. But, if the blood supply to the kidney is blocked, the kidney can secrete renin without consulting the brain.

High Blood Pressure

The normal regulation of blood pressure is complicated. In about 10% to 15% of adults, the system of regulation goes off a bit, and the blood pressure becomes persistently elevated. This is what we call *high blood pressure* or *hypertension*. Hypertension means a persistently abnormal increase of blood pressure due to the malfunction of one or several of the factors responsible for maintaining normal blood pressure (discussed below). We must clear up a common misunderstanding here. *Hypertension does* not *mean that a person is "hyper" or "tense" in the sense of being nervous.* Usually, high blood pressure has nothing to do with stress or nervous tension. The reasons for high blood pressure are discussed in detail below.

But where does high blood pressure begin and normal blood pressure end? Even the authorities in this area do not always agree on the exact number at which health ends and disease starts. Most agree that blood pressure is normal up to 140/90 mm Hg. Above that level, the increase of blood pressure leads to important increases in the risk of heart disease, stroke, kidney damage and damage to the large blood vessels of the body. As one might expect, the risk increases as the blood pressure rises.

A practical definition of high blood pressure is the level at which treatment to lower the blood pressure does more good than harm. Chapter 3 provides details about this level.

Low Blood Pressure

Although this book is about high blood pressure, it is difficult not to mention low blood pressure. If you do not have low blood pressure, you can skip to the next section.

In general, we do not define low blood pressure by a number, as we do for high blood pressure; rather we rely on the presence of symptoms to show if there is a problem. You may have heard someone say that they are tired as a result of low blood pressure. Indeed, low blood pressure may lead to symptoms such as fatigue. Fortunately, the complications for low blood pressure are not as severe as those for high blood pressure. On the other hand, when our blood pressure gets too low, the brain does not receive enough blood, and we get dizzy. If this continues or becomes more severe, we can faint. This is most likely to occur when we stand up. This certainly can be a nuisance and can sometimes have serious consequences, for example, if we fall and break a bone. There are several treatments for this problem; you should consult your doctor if you become very lightheaded when you stand.

What Causes High Blood Pressure?

If you have high blood pressure, there are many factors that could have caused it. However, in most cases (95%), when we test a person to find out why their blood pressure is high, none of the factors that we can measure seems to be upset.

In some cases — about 1 in 20 — we can find the cause, such as an endocrine gland secreting an excessive amount of a hormone, or a decreasing blood supply to the kidneys. In these cases, we refer to the high blood pressure as *secondary hypertension*. Some of the causes of secondary hypertension can be cured and some cannot.

Table 1-1 lists the causes of hypertension, which are arranged from the most to the least frequent. Recalling that only 1 of every 20 people with hypertension has one of the secondary causes, some of them are rare indeed. We will discuss each of them in order.

Essential hypertension. When we cannot determine the cause for high blood pressure, we call it essential hyperten-

Table 1-1: Causes of Hypertension (in decreasing order of occurrence)
1. Essential (unknown cause, 95% of patients)
2. Diseases of the kidney
3. Decreased blood supply to the kidneys (renovascular)
4. Primary aldosteronism
5. Coarctation (narrowing) of the aorta
6. Cushing's syndrome
7. Oral contraceptives
8. Pheochromocytoma

sion. The vast majority of people with high blood pressure have *essential hypertension*. No doubt, there are underlying causes for essential hypertension, such as heredity, but we do not understand them as yet. Thus medical science is still faced with an enigma about a disease that affects over 10% of the world's adult population. (In children, an underlying cause is more likely to be found.) On the brighter side, even without understanding some aspects of the disease, we do know how to treat high blood pressure and, as discussed in Chapter 3, we know that lowering the blood pressure by treatment prevents most of its complications.

Diseases of the kidney. The kidney plays an important role in the regulation of blood pressure, and it is natural that some of the diseases of the kidney affect blood pressure adversely. As the function of a diseased kidney declines, the blood pressure usually becomes elevated. Unfortunately, there is often little that can be done to cure chronic kidney disease. However, if the blood pressure does become elevated, it must — and can — be treated effectively to avoid further damage to the kidneys and other organs from the high blood pressure itself.

Decreased blood supply to the kidneys. Hypertension that is caused by decreased blood supply to the kidneys is called *renovascular hypertension*. Usually, each kidney receives its blood supply from a major artery, called the *renal artery*. If this artery becomes narrowed, reducing the blood supply to the kidney, the kidney secretes renin to raise the blood pressure so the flow of blood can be restored. Unfortunately, the pressure is raised throughout the whole system and the result is hypertension.

There are two main causes of narrowing of the arteries to the kidneys. First, and most common, is when arteries become narrowed by *atherosclerosis* or "hardening of the arteries". This is more common in late middle age and onward. The second cause is called *fibromuscular hyperplasia*. This occurs mainly in young women during their childbearing years and may be aggravated by pregnancy. In either case, the condition often can be treated surgically by bypassing the affected artery. This procedure is a forerunner of the now famous coronary artery bypass. More recently, a less difficult method, *angioplasty*, has been developed for opening the artery. This is done by stretching or dilating the inside of the artery, using a catheter with a balloon at its tip. The catheter is a hollow tube that is inserted in a major artery in the groin and moved up the artery to the opening of the artery to the kidney, the renal artery. The tip of the catheter is then moved to the site of the narrowing of the renal artery. The balloon is then inflated through the catheter, stretching the renal artery at the narrowed section. Usually the procedure can be done in hospital in less than an hour and the patient can go home the same or next day.

Primary aldosteronism. *Aldosterone* is a hormone secreted by the adrenal glands. It plays a role in the balance of fluid and salt in the body. If too much of the hormone is secreted, for example, by a tumour in the adrenal gland, too much salt is retained in the body. This has the effect of elevating blood pressure. If the excess secretion of aldosterone is due to a single tumour that can be removed, surgery is usually the treatment of choice. However, if both adrenal glands are involved, the treatment is usually a medication, such as *spironolactone*, that blocks the effect of the aldosterone.

Coarctation of the aorta. *Coarctation* is a medical word for narrowing. Narrowing of the aorta, the major artery leading away from the heart, results in decreased blood supply to the lower part of the body including the kidneys. The kidneys try to overcome this problem by secreting renin, which raises the blood pressure. Coarctation is generally a problem with which a person is born; it causes hypertension early in life. The treatment is to remove the narrowing surgically.

Cushing's syndrome. *Cushing's syndrome* is a disorder in which the adrenal glands secrete too much cortisol. This is a complex disorder. Its management usually requires collaboration between specialists in endocrine disease and surgery.

Oral contraceptives. *Oral contraceptives* that contain estrogen can raise the blood pressure, sometimes to the level of hypertension. Often the blood pressure will return to normal when the birth control medication is stopped. If you are a woman on oral contraceptives and have high blood pressure, you should be sure to remind your doctor of this. Estrogen levels also rise in pregnancy and sometimes cause elevated pressures. Postmenopausal estrogen therapy is less likely to raise blood pressure. For more information, see Chapter 14.

Pheochromocytoma. This exotic-sounding problem is due to yet another disorder of the adrenal glands. The central part of the adrenal glands, called the *medulla*, secretes the hormones *adrenaline* and *noradrenaline*. If this part of the gland becomes hyperactive, then the blood pressure becomes elevated. Often, the excess secretion comes in bursts and causes characteristic symptoms including a fast, pounding heartbeat, headache, sweating and trembling. Unless you have bouts of this nature *with all the symptoms at the same time*, you are unlikely to have pheochromocytoma. Most of the tumours that cause pheochromocytoma are benign and can be removed surgically. Sometimes the tumour is malignant and develops, or has spread, outside the adrenal glands by the time it is discovered and cannot be treated surgically.

Other causes of hypertension. There are some other rare causes of hypertension. First, excess ingestion of licorice can have an effect similar to increased aldosterone (see above) and can raise the blood pressure. The solution for this problem is obvious! Second, other endocrine problems such as *acromegaly* (excess secretion of growth hormone from the pituitary gland in the head) and *hyperparathyroidism* (excess secretion of hormone from the parathyroid glands in the neck) can cause elevated blood pressure. Third, hereditary diseases such as *polycystic kidney disease* cause hypertension. Fourth, it is likely that heredity determines a person's response to salt in the diet or psychological stress. These are discussed in more detail in Chapters 4 and 5, respectively.

How High Blood Pressure Affects the Body

High blood pressure — if untreated for long periods of time — can cause damage to the arteries of the body and to the organs they supply, especially the heart, brain and kidneys (Fig. 1-2).

Before going into the details, we must emphasize that most of the bad effects caused by high blood pressure can be prevented if the blood pressure is brought down to normal by treatment. It is also important to understand that factors

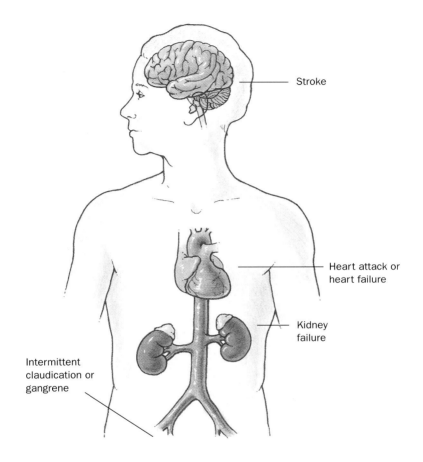

Stroke

Heart attack or
heart failure

Kidney
failure

Intermittent
claudication or
gangrene

Figure 1-2: Consequences of uncontrolled hypertension

such as smoking, high cholesterol and diabetes can cause similar damage to the body and that these factors should also be controlled.

The heart. Like any muscle in the body forced to do extra work, the heart becomes bigger when it has to pump against higher pressure. Although the heart can stand a high pressure for quite a long time, eventually, over many years, it will

17

begin to fail. When this happens, fluid from the blood backs up into the lungs and the lungs become "waterlogged". Because the heart has difficulty pumping blood to the muscles when they need extra oxygen for exercise or work, a person will feel short of breath. At first, the shortness of breath comes on only while a person is active. Eventually, breathing becomes difficult even during rest. The technical term for this problem is *congestive heart failure*.

The heart also has its own blood supply through vessels called the *coronary arteries*. The arteries to the heart can be hardened and narrowed in the same way that arteries to other organs are damaged. (This is discussed in detail in the next section.) When the coronary arteries become too narrow to carry enough oxygen for the heart to do its work, a person experiences the sensation of pressure, tightness or heaviness in the chest, arm or jaw that lasts for about 5 minutes and goes away with rest. This sort of pain is called *angina pectoris*, or *angina* for short. At first, this sensation comes on only with exercise or strenuous work. Later, it can come on with very little activity or with excitement or emotional upset.

Although the discomfort of angina is a warning of too little blood supply to the heart, no permanent damage is done by it. Often, just lowering the blood pressure can reduce the work of the heart enough to relieve the angina. However, if the blood supply to a part of the heart is blocked even more, permanent damage is done to the heart muscle. This is called a heart attack or *myocardial infarction* or "coronary" or coronary thrombosis. This is usually signalled by longer chest pain than that caused by angina (typically, at least 15 minutes and often much longer) as well as nausea and sweating. A heart attack can be fatal but, if a person can get to the hospital in time, the chances for a good recovery are high.

The arteries. As times goes on, all humans develop hardening of the arteries whether or not they have high blood pressure. Hardening of the arteries is due to the walls of arteries becoming thicker and less elastic. The increased thickening causes narrowing of the artery, eventually blocking blood flow. High blood pressure causes an increase in the rate at which hardening of the arteries occurs.

The arteries of the body do not all narrow at the same rate. The effects of narrowing of the arteries depend on which organs are fed by the narrowed arteries. For example, as we just discussed, if any artery to the heart muscle becomes blocked, the result is a heart attack. If an artery to the brain is blocked, then a *stroke* occurs. If the blood supply to the kidneys is blocked by this process, then *nephrosclerosis* occurs with the kidneys becoming shrunken and eventually failing. The arteries to the legs can also be affected. When these arteries become narrowed, cramps occur in the legs during walking, similar in nature to the "cramp" of the heart with angina, but called *intermittent claudication*. As with angina, this pain also goes away in a few minutes with rest. However, if the narrowing of the arteries of the legs becomes very severe, pain occurs even at rest. Eventually, the tissues of the leg, starting with the toes, die. This is called *gangrene*.

Narrowing of the arteries to the bowel also gives rise to cramps — in the stomach area or just below — a condition called *abdominal angina*. Complete blockage of the blood supply to the bowel causes bleeding from the bowel and usually infection sets in, causing a person to be very sick.

If the blood pressure elevation is mild, the increase in the rate of hardening of the arteries is not great. Usually, the blood pressure must be elevated for many years before there are adverse effects. Recall that if the blood pressure is brought back to normal by treatment, the risk of complications is reduced.

If the blood pressure is severely elevated for a period of time, then the consequences come sooner and are usually much worse. Rather than gradual narrowing of the vessels, severely elevated pressure can cause the blood vessels to burst. When blood leaks out of a blood vessel it is called a *hemorrhage*. Hemorrhage into the brain causes a serious, often fatal stroke. Severely elevated pressure can also cause the largest artery of the body, the aorta, to bulge and even burst. The bulge is called an aneurysm and the bursting process is called a *dissection*.

Fortunately, serious blood pressure elevations are uncommon. When they do happen, often there are warning signs before these severe problems occur. The warnings of severely elevated blood pressure include headache, nosebleeds, blurred vision, and sometimes chest pains or pains in the abdomen. Again, these complications are unlikely to occur unless high blood pressure is neglected and left untreated for a prolonged period.

The brain. Some of the effects of hypertension on the brain have already been mentioned. A person with high blood pressure, particularly when it is longstanding and uncontrolled, has a much greater risk of stroke (about seven times the risk, on average, if the high blood pressure is untreated) than a person with normal blood pressure.

A stroke can occur in three ways. First, hardening of the arteries can lead to the inside lining of the larger arteries becoming unsmooth and cracked. Small clots or bits of debris can collect on these roughened areas. They can then break off, becoming stuck in smaller arteries "down stream". This blocks the blood supply, resulting in a stroke. The broken-off bits are called *emboli*, and this type of event is called an *embolic stroke*. Second, the narrowing in the larger arteries can be so great that the blood supply is blocked in them. This is either a direct effect of the narrowing or due to a clot forming in the narrowed artery. The result is an *atherothrombotic stroke*. Finally, if the pressure is high enough, an artery can actually burst, causing a hemorrhage into the brain, a *hemorrhagic stroke*. Although hemorrhagic strokes are usually the most severe, they are fortunately also the rarest. Even better, the occurrence of hemorrhagic stroke has been decreased by blood pressure-lowering treatment more than the other kinds.

If the blood pressure is severely elevated, then the blood vessels can break down quickly. This results in leakage of fluid and blood cells into the brain (without frank hemorrhage) and leads to symptoms of very severe headache and fatigue. Because the skull, in which the brain sits, does not allow any expansion, the leakage of fluid into the brain increases the pressure inside the skull and can damage the brain directly.

The good news is that over the last three decades the rate of all these complications has decreased dramatically. This is the result of the control of high blood pressure with modern treatments. High blood pressure does increase the risk of stroke, but the likelihood of you having a stroke depends on the level of blood pressure elevation. If your blood pressure is controlled, you are at no greater risk of a stroke than someone with normal blood pressure.

Although the treatment of hypertension plays an important role in stroke prevention, other options such as aspirin, blood thinners (anticoagulants) and surgery involving the arteries in the neck also need to be considered by patients and their physicians.

The kidneys. Not only can the kidneys cause high blood pressure (see above), but high blood pressure (due to whatever cause) can also cause kidney damage.

High blood pressure reduces the blood flow to the kidneys. This is thought to be due to an increase in the resistance in the small arteries of the kidney. The hardening of the arteries caused by the high blood pressure also reduces blood flow to the kidneys. Initially, the kidney's job of filtering the blood for wastes is not affected. If the hypertension becomes more severe or has a greater duration, there is eventually further reduction in blood flow to the kidneys.

In addition to the effect on blood flow, very high blood pressure directly damages the filtering system in the kidneys. The result is that the kidneys are no longer able to filter out wastes from the blood stream, and these consequently build up in the body. The more severe the hypertension, the more direct the damage to the filtering system.

Fortunately, kidney complications are the easiest ones to prevent with high blood pressure treatment. These days, we hardly ever see people with kidney failure due to hypertension.

Death. Hypertension has been called the "silent killer" because it usually causes few symptoms until a considerable amount of damage has been done. The damage can then be fatal in the form of a heart attack, stroke or, less often, bleeding from a burst artery, or kidney failure.

What Can Be Done To Prevent These Complications?

Because most people with high blood pressure have their blood pressure elevation detected before any complications occur and because modern treatments for high blood pressure can bring the blood pressure back to normal, the term "silent killer" is rapidly becoming outdated.

Unfortunately, there are some people whose blood pressure elevation goes undetected because they seldom see a doctor. There are also patients who drop out of treatment or fail to take the treatment that has been prescribed for them. This is a tragic situation as elevated blood pressure can truly be a cause of early death. It has been estimated that untreated moderate hypertension reduces one's life span by an average of more than 16 years. If life does indeed begin at 40, hypertension can cut short the best part of your life. If you have high blood pressure, make sure you get good treatment for it! Ways in which to do this are discussed in the rest of this book, particularly in Chapter 15.

DIAGNOSTIC TESTS

Richard A. Reeves, MD, and

Martin J. Bass, MD, MSc

This chapter has four aims. First, we will describe how blood pressure (BP) is measured. Second, we will consider how these measurements are used to make the diagnosis of high blood pressure. Third, we will look at some questions your doctor may ask and tests he or she may order if you do have high blood pressure. Finally, we answer some common questions that our patients have asked us.

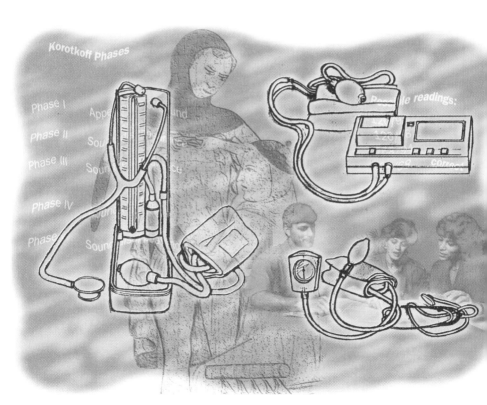

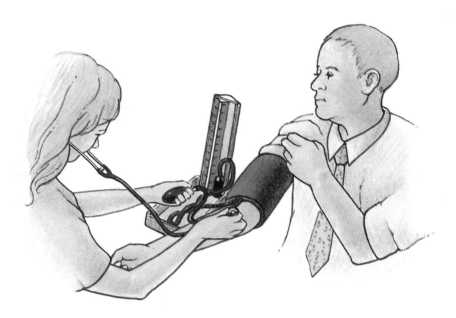

Figure 2-1: Measuring blood pressure

How Is Blood Pressure Measured?

The measurement of blood pressure is simple, quick and virtually painless. A properly sized cuff placed around the arm is
filled with enough air to squeeze the artery. This temporarily
stops the flow of blood. As the air is slowly released, the doctor
or nurse — or you — listens with a stethoscope as the blood
starts to rush through the artery (Fig.2-1).

The first tapping sound heard is the *systolic blood pressure*.
The systolic blood pressure is the maximum pressure produced
when the heart beats and pumps blood into the arteries. The
pressure is expressed as millimetres of mercury, or in symbols,
"mm Hg". A normal systolic blood pressure usually ranges
between 100 to 140 mm Hg. A systolic blood pressure
between 140 and 159 mm Hg is borderline; if the systolic
blood pressure is 160 mm Hg or greater, it is called "elevated".

The second measure used for diagnosis is the *diastolic blood
pressure*. As more air is released from the cuff, a point is

reached where the artery is fully open. At this point, the blood flows smoothly and the tapping sound over the artery disappears. The pressure when this last sound disappears is called the diastolic blood pressure. The diastolic blood pressure represents the pressure in the arteries between heartbeats. The diastolic blood pressure normally ranges between 60 to 90 mm Hg. A diastolic blood pressure consistently 90 mm Hg or greater is considered elevated.

For convenience, these two readings are written down together. For example, "130/80" indicates a blood pressure of 130 mm Hg systolic and 80 mm Hg diastolic.

Blood pressures taken when you are lying, sitting or standing are usually very similar. However, some people, particularly the elderly and diabetics, may have much lower pressures when they stand up. Also, some drugs lower standing blood pressure more than lying blood pressure. In these situations, the pressure is often measured both while lying and standing. Many doctors feel that the most useful blood pressure measurement is one taken while sitting quietly, without talking, because it represents the usual way most of us spend our daytime hours.

No matter which position you are in, you must be comfortable and have your arm supported. If the arm is unsupported, the arm muscles have to work, and this raises the blood pressure readings. Support can be given by the doctor's or nurse's hand, or by resting your arm on a table or the arm of a chair. Also, it is not uncommon to find up to a 5 mm Hg difference between the two arms. The custom is to use the arm with the higher blood pressure for all subsequent visits.

What Is the Role of Home Blood Pressure Measurement ?

Certain people have consistently lower blood pressure at home than at their doctor's office. Some people also find it helpful to see the effect of their medications on their blood pressure. In addition, some doctors believe it is easier to adjust medications and to help people follow their treatments if blood pressures are taken between visits as well as at the clinic. If you are interested in purchasing a blood pressure kit for your own use, see Chapter 15. However, be aware that the diagnosis of high blood pressure is based on the office blood pressure. At present, the role of home or self-monitored blood pressure remains unclear, and further research is needed.

All people doing self-monitoring should have proper training in the method and need to have their machines checked periodically for accuracy. It helps to have a physician or nurse available to contact. In some patients self-monitoring of blood pressure may result in excess concern about the usual peaks of blood pressure and may increase anxieties about health. It is important to understand that blood pressure varies with time in everyone. This means the blood pressure could be 156/92 mm Hg at one time and 132/86 just a few minutes later. This variability is normal. The level of blood pressure used to decide about treatment is based on the average of several readings, not any single reading.

You may be able to obtain additional readings in other ways, too. If a nurse visits your home regularly or if you can see a nurse at your place of work, have her/him check your blood pressure and write down the readings with the date and time so you can show these readings to your doctor. However, we do not recommend using machines available in public places such as shopping centres. These are often quite inaccurate.

What Is Ambulatory Blood Pressure Monitoring ?

Portable automatic blood pressure measuring devices are now available through some doctors' offices. These can record blood pressures many times throughout the day. A typical blood pressure cuff is worn, and a small pump inflates and deflates the cuff automatically. These machines are no larger than a paperback book and are worn on the belt or a shoulder strap. They are reasonably comfortable to wear and don't usually disrupt the daily routine or sleep. Information is stored in the unit's memory and later transferred to a computer for printout. With these machines, an average blood pressure can be determined during many different activities. Of interest, average ambulatory blood pressure during the day is about 5 mm Hg lower than the office blood pressure.

Ambulatory blood pressure monitoring is still mainly a research tool. It may be useful in patients who have only borderline pressure elevation, or if "White Coat Syndrome" is suspected. In this condition, blood pressure is elevated in the physician's office but is lower elsewhere or even normal. However, only further research will clarify whether a patient with hypertension in the office but a normal ambulatory blood pressure can safely go without treatment. For now, both ambulatory blood pressure and home blood pressure are best viewed as providing special pieces of information that are sometimes used in deciding whether an elevated office blood pressure requires treatment or not.

How Is High Blood Pressure Diagnosed?

Does one elevated blood pressure reading mean that you have "high blood pressure"? No! As we mentioned, blood pressure varies continuously. There are many reasons for pressures to be high at any one time. Pressures taken just after exercise or when you are upset may be higher as a temporary response to the situation. A blood pressure that remains high after 5 minutes of sitting quietly is more important. Even then, just the situation of having one's blood pressure taken can elevate the reading. To overcome this, your physician may measure your blood pressure twice or more during a visit and record only the lowest pressure.

Medical authorities agree that a minimum of two elevated blood pressure readings taken on at least two or three different days are needed to make the diagnosis of high blood pressure or *hypertension.* Furthermore, research shows that blood pressure taken in the doctor's office may continue to drop for up to 6 months. Because of this, the Canadian Hypertension Society recommends that, *for people whose diastolic blood pressure appears only mildly elevated, the diagnosis of "high blood pressure" should be based on at least three blood pressure measurements over a period of 6 months.* This period may be shortened if the blood pressure is moderately elevated or if there is any evidence of damage from the high blood pressure.

Unfortunately, there are many people who believe they have high blood pressure because they've had one elevated blood pressure reading, even though readings after that time have been normal. In fact, a recent survey showed that more people with normal readings *thought* they had high blood pressure than there were people who actually had high blood pressure. If you are not on antihypertensive medication and your blood pressure at your doctor's office is usually normal (less than 140/90 mm Hg), then you do not have hypertension!

When Is Systolic Blood Pressure Important ?

A systolic blood pressure repeatedly 160 mm Hg or greater with a diastolic blood pressure below 90 mm Hg is called *isolated systolic hypertension.* Elevated systolic pressure with or without elevated diastolic pressure occurs mostly in the elderly. Treating elevated systolic pressure has recently been proved to decrease the risk of heart disease and stroke, at least for persons age 60 and older. This is an important new finding.

The Doctor's Investigation of High Blood Pressure

Once the doctor has made certain that you really have high blood pressure, he/she will investigate further (Fig. 2-2). The investigation involves four main steps:

1. An interview about your medical history, current health and related activities (Table 2-1),
2. A physical examination (Table 2-2),
3. Routine tests (Table 2-3), and
4. Other tests may be done (Table 2-4).

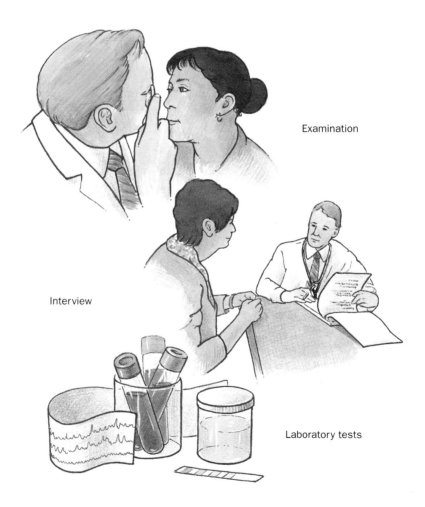

Examination

Interview

Laboratory tests

Figure 2-2: Diagnosing high blood pressure

Table 2-1: The Doctor's Interview Regarding High BP

Question	Looking for	Why?
1. Are you taking any medications?	Birth control pill, estrogens, cold remedies, diet pills	Easily removed cause
2. Do you eat licorice daily?	Large amount of licorice	Easily removed cause
3. How much alcohol do you drink per day?	Average of more than two drinks per day	Can cause elevated BP
4. Do you restrict your salt intake?	Salt intake	Reduction may lower BP
5. Have you been under recent stress?	Recent stress may raise BP	May need to measure BP at less stressful time
6. Have you recently gained or lost weight?	Recent weight change	Overweight causes high BP; unplanned weight loss suggests thyroid or adrenal medulla hyperactivity
7. Have you ever had kidney problems?	Kidney infection, kidney diseases, stones, bleeding, trauma	Can cause hypertension
8. Have you ever had a heart problem or stroke ?	History of heart attack or stroke?	Effect of BP on body
9. Any transient loss of vision, numbness or paralysis?	Warning of stroke	Effect of BP on brain
10. Do you have leg pains when walking?	Pain that stops with rest	Arteries of legs affected

(*Continued next page*)

11. Have family members had heart attacks or strokes?	Family history	Increased risk of heart attack or stroke
12. Do you smoke?	Regular smoking	Increased chance of heart and artery trouble and stroke
13. Do you exercise?	Healthy habits	Reduce overall risk
14. Do you know your cholesterol?	Elevation	Additional risk
15. Do you restrict fat?	Good diet	Lower heart disease risk

Table 2-2: The Doctor's Physical Examination

Examination	Looking for	As Evidence of
Height, weight	Overweight	Excess weight as possible cause, increased risk
Look into eyes	Twisted blood vessels, red and white patches	Blood vessels affected by BP
Listen to abdomen, neck, groin	High-pitched sounds	Narrowing of artery to kidney, brain or leg
Look at skin	Violet stretch marks on abdomen	Adrenal hyperactivity
BP in both arms, or take pulse at wrist and groin, or BP taken in the leg	Difference between arms, or delay in pulse at groin or lowered pressure in the leg	Coarctation; important for future BP measurement
Listen to heart	Abnormal heart sounds	Heart enlargement or failure from high BP

Listen to chest	Fluid in lungs	Heart failure from high BP
Feel the neck pulses; and thyroid gland	Narrowed arteries; or thyroid disease	Blood vessels affected by BP; may raise BP
Feel the feet	Poor circulation; swelling	Blood vessels affected by BP; heart failure

Table 2-3: Routine Laboratory Tests for High BP

Test	Looking for	As Evidence of
Urine sample	Protein, cells, sugar (glucose)	Kidney problems, diabetes mellitus
Blood potassium	Low potassium	Overactive adrenal gland
Blood creatinine or urea	Elevation	Kidney problems
Electrocardiogram (ECG/EKG)	Effect of BP on heart	Heart enlargement or previous heart damage
Chest x-ray (optional)	Heart enlargement, fluid	Effect of BP on heart, heart failure

Table 2-4: Other Tests That May Be Done

Test	Looking for	As Evidence of
Blood cholesterol	High cholesterol	Increased risk of heart disease
Blood sugar	High sugar	Diabetes mellitus

(Continued next page)

Echocardiogram	Enlarged heart or abnormality of heart function	Effect of BP on heart
24-hour urine	Elevated VMA or metanephrines, cortisol or aldosterone; high protein; excess salt	Overactive adrenal gland; kidney problems; high sodium intake
Renal scan (renogram), intravenous pyelogram (rarely)	Reduced size or functioning of kidneys	Kidney problem as result or cause of hypertension
Renal vein renin test	High renin output from one kidney	Narrowed artery to one kidney
Renal arteriogram	Narrowing of renal artery	Can raise BP; may be curable
Home BP	Lower blood pressure at home	Over-reactive BP in doctor's office
Ambulatory blood pressure monitor	BP changes with time and activity during daily activity	Accurate measure of BP over 24 hours
Blood count	Anemia	May increase systolic BP

Each time the doctor does one of the above steps, he/she is trying to find the answer to at least one of the following three questions:

1. What is the *cause* of the high blood pressure?
2. Has the high blood pressure had any lasting *effect* on your body?
3. Are there any *other factors* that may increase your chance

of having a stroke, heart problems or other complications of high blood pressure?

Finding a cause for the high blood pressure may allow partial or complete cure. If the elevated blood pressure has affected your body or you have other factors that increase the risk of a complication, it may be important to start treatment at lower levels of elevated blood pressure. Also, if you do have other untreated risk factors, these will need to be attended to. We will look into each of these three questions in the sections that follow.

What Is the Cause of Your High Blood Pressure?

In about 95 of 100 cases no clear cause of high blood pressure can be found even after a thorough investigation. As explained in Chapter 1, this is called *primary* or *essential* hypertension (Fig.2-3). In only about one to two of 100 cases is a treatable cause found. In the rest of the cases in which a cause can be found, it cannot be cured — although the blood pressure can almost always be controlled.

The most easily treated causes of elevated blood pressure can all be discovered by simple questions or examinations (Fig.2-4). Here are some questions that your doctor may ask:

Are You Taking Any Medications?

Some drugs, both prescription and nonprescription, increase blood pressure. By stopping them, the blood pressure often returns to normal. The most commonly used drugs that can elevate blood pressure are birth control pills and other "hormone pills" that contain estrogen. Cold or sinus remedies or allergy tablets that contain decongestants can constrict the blood vessels and can occasionally raise blood pressure. A similar effect is seen with some diet pills and herbal remedies. Nonsteroidal anti-inflammatory drugs (NSAIDs) such as ibuprofen, commonly used to relieve arthritis, can also raise blood pressure.

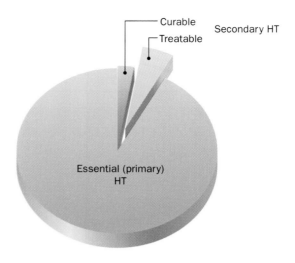

Curable
Treatable
Secondary HT
Essential (primary) HT

Figure 2-3: Essential (primary) hypertension

Licorice, Alcohol or Salt Intake? Any Change in Your Weight?

Things that you eat and drink can affect your blood pressure. Only the rare person eats (or drinks, in herbal tea) a lot of licorice every day, but that is easily remedied. The more alcohol one drinks (above two drinks per day), the higher the blood pressure. This rise in pressure is quickly reversed by cutting back on alcohol. Some people's blood pressure is "salt sensitive" (see Chapter 5). High blood pressure is also related to being overweight.

Have You Been under Stress Recently?

A stressful situation such as a problem at work, a financial crisis, or family troubles can raise your blood pressure *temporarily*. If the doctor finds that you are under stress, he may choose to have you come back at a less stressful time to recheck your blood pressure.

We must note here that many people think that high blood pressure is a "stress" disease and that every person who is anxious or under stress has high blood pressure. This is seldom the case. People who feel stressed may have high blood pressure,

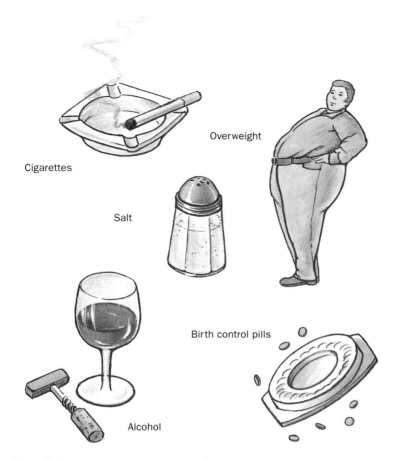

Cigarettes

Overweight

Salt

Birth control pills

Alcohol

Figure 2-4: Reversible environmental factors

but this is not often due to the stress itself. On the other hand, people who feel relaxed can still have high blood pressure. The only way to tell is to measure the blood pressure!

Have You Had Any Problems with Your Kidneys ?
As explained in Chapter 1, the kidneys play an important role in controlling your blood pressure. Since kidney problems may lead to high blood pressure, your doctor will look for:

Chronic renal disease. Chronic kidney disease stands as the most frequent rare cause of high blood pressure. The doctor will inquire about chronic kidney and urinary infections, kidney injury from accidents or kidney stones. He/she will examine your urine for protein and cells that should not be there. He/she will also take blood tests for *creatinine* or *urea* as indicators of how well the kidneys are working.

Narrowing of the artery to the kidney ("renal artery stenosis"). If the blood supply to a kidney is reduced because of a partial blockage, the kidney will respond by demanding a higher blood pressure. Blood flowing through the narrowed artery can make a noise that can be heard through the doctor's stethoscope. If he/she hears this noise when listening over your abdomen, he may then order a *renal* scan, a test that involves the injection of a small — and safe — amount of radioactive dye and then lying beneath a scanner that "sees" the dye as it is taken up by the kidneys. Another similar test is the *intravenous pyelogram* or *IVP*. This involves the injection of a small amount of dye or *contrast* that shows up on an x-ray when the dye enters the kidneys.

If a blocked artery to the kidney is still suspected after the initial tests, then an x-ray picture can be taken of the artery to the kidney. This x-ray is called an *arteriogram* or *angiogram*. A small tube is inserted through an artery in the groin and moved inside the artery until it is near the kidney. X-ray dye is then injected. As the dye flows through the artery to the kidney, an x-ray movie will reveal any blockage or narrowing.

As final proof that the kidney with a narrowed artery is causing the high blood pressure, a *renal vein renin test* may be performed. Renin is a hormone produced by the kidney to raise blood pressure. If one kidney is causing the high blood pressure, it may overproduce renin. This is measured through a small tube inserted into a groin vein to reach the vein leaving each kidney.

Could You Have "Coarctation of the Aorta"?
This is a narrowing of the main artery leaving the heart, which reduces the flow of blood to the legs. The clue the doctor

looks for is a delay between the pulse of your wrist and groin, or a higher blood pressure in your arm than in your leg.

Do You Have Any Problems with Your Adrenal Glands ?

Primary aldosteronism. The adrenals are small glands that secrete hormones from their location atop each kidney. An overactive adrenal gland can produce an excess of the hormone *aldosterone*, which raises blood pressure. Low potassium in the blood is a clue.

Adrenal hyperactivity (Cushing's syndrome). If the adrenal glands produce too much of the hormone *cortisone*, the blood pressure will be raised. The clue to this disease is unusual weight gain on the upper back and abdomen. Distinctive violet-coloured stretch marks may develop on the abdomen. Blood or urine testing will reveal excess cortisone.

Pheochromocytoma. The cause of high blood pressure here is a tumour of the central part of the adrenal gland, the adrenal medulla. The clues come from the medical history. Persons with this problem complain of attacks of headache, sweating, tremor and heart palpitations. If you report these symptoms, the doctor will ask you to collect your urine for 24 hours. This is then analyzed for chemicals secreted by the tumor. If this test is positive, then special x-rays are done to locate the tumour, which can often be removed by surgery.

Has the Blood Pressure Affected Your Body ?

As discussed more fully in Chapter 1, if your blood pressure is very high or high for a long time, it can affect several bodily organs. If the doctor finds such effects of high blood pressure, this is important knowledge when deciding about treatment.

When the heart works against higher pressure it becomes larger. Important enlargement leads to changes in the *electrocar-*

diogram, or *ECG (EKG)*, and the *echocardiogram* (ultrasound of the heart). A chest x-ray is a less sensitive way to show increases in heart size. If the heart muscle is overworked for a very long time, fluid may back up into the lungs. This is called *congestive heart failure*. The fluid is easily heard over the lungs with a stethoscope and can be seen on the chest x-ray.

A second area of the body to be affected is the kidney. Prolonged high blood pressure can wear out the kidneys. This can be detected by a simple blood test. A 24-hour urine collection is often added for more information.

High blood pressure can also affect the blood vessels. By looking into the eye with an ophthalmoscope, the doctor can see what is happening to the blood vessels in the body. With severe hypertension, the blood vessels become narrowed and twisted. The vessels can also leak fluid or blood that can be seen as white or red patches on the back of the eye. The doctor will also examine the large blood vessels of the body for narrowing or enlargement due to high blood pressure.

Is Your Chance of Having Complications Increased by Factors besides High Blood pressure ?

Since high blood pressure is treated primarily to lower your chance of having a stroke or heart trouble, your doctor must know about anything else that could increase your chance of having either of these problems. Because your chances of a stroke or heart trouble are higher if members of your close family have had either of these, if you smoke, or if you have diabetes or increased cholesterol, the doctor will check these as well.

Questions and Answers

People with high blood pressure usually have many questions about their condition. We will answer some of the more common ones.

1. Why is my blood pressure sometimes higher when I feel fine and I have been taking all my medicines as prescribed?

Blood pressure is constantly going up and down as we go about our activities. As we mentioned earlier, it is quite usual for the diastolic pressure to vary by as much as 10 to 15 mm Hg, even over a few minutes. If we are rushed or anxious it may be higher for a short time. Sometimes taking a new medication may cause the pressure to go up. Talking while the blood pressure is being taken can also raise the pressure. Smoking may raise blood pressure briefly. The blood pressure will also be elevated somewhat if the pressure is taken when the arm is not comfortably supported. Finally, the blood pressure in any person may increase over time so their medication must be increased.

2. When the doctor is trying to find out whether the high blood pressure has affected your body, why doesn't he/she always ask about headaches?

Unless it is very high, high blood pressure has *no* symptoms. Persons with mildly to moderately high blood pressure have the same number and types of headaches as people with normal blood pressure.

3. Is there a difference between a blood pressure measured with a mercury sphygmomanometer and one with a round dial (aneroid) or a digital electronic machine?

Mercury column instruments provide the most accurate and dependable measurement of blood pressure. There is little that can go wrong with these simple devices. The dial and electronic machines are generally easier to use, but need to be checked for accuracy regularly. A properly calibrated dial (or electronic) machine will show the same blood pressure as a mercury device. Chapter 15 has more information about blood pressure machines.

4. Do I have high blood pressure if only my systolic or diastolic pressure is high?

If *either* your systolic blood pressure *or* diastolic blood pressure stays elevated (at or above 140 mm Hg systolic or 90 mm Hg diastolic or both) on three different occasions over 6 months, then you have high blood pressure or hypertension.

We must note here that there is not full agreement among doctors on the need to treat mild hypertension in all patients. If the systolic blood pressure is between 140 and 159 mm Hg or the diastolic blood pressure is between 90 and 99 mm Hg and there is no evidence of damage to the heart, brain, kidney or major arteries, then other factors will be taken into account in reaching a decision. These factors include other risks such as smoking, male gender, diabetes, cholesterol and family history of cardiovascular disease.

CHAPTER 3

BENEFITS OF TREATMENT

David L. Sackett, MD, MSc

You have learned from the earlier chapters in this book that high blood pressure is bad for you. It shortens your life and increases your chances of having a heart attack, a stroke, permanent damage to your vision, damage to your kidneys, or ballooning (aneurysm) of your biggest artery (the aorta). You have also learned that high blood pressure is almost always "silent" until you have one of these complications. Almost everyone with high blood pressure has no symptoms until complications set in.

This chapter will answer the question: "Why treat high blood pressure?" The simple answer is: "Because treating high blood pressure decreases your chances of suffering one of its complications!" However, because this answer means that you will have to take medicine, follow a fairly strict diet, or change your lifestyle even though you may feel perfectly well, you deserve an explanation.

How To Tell Whether Treatment Does More Good Than Harm

How can we tell if a treatment should be prescribed by doctors and accepted by patients? How can we know that the treatment does more good than harm? After all, it wasn't all that long ago that doctors prescribed opium for diabetes. In fact, several decades ago this was recommended by William Osler, one of the world's most famous doctors. The first U. S. president was also a victim of bad medical advice. He had a severe sore throat and was prescribed "blood letting". This was a common medical practice in his day and consisted of taking several units of his blood over a few days to "let the bad humours out". The result was fatal. The treatment was far worse than the disease!

In modern times, health scientists have developed powerful methods for proving whether a new treatment does more good than harm. Rather than relying on testimonials or the advice of famous physicians, this modern health science insists that new treatments be tested in special experiments called "randomized clinical trials".

A randomized clinical trial (Figure 3-1) uses a system that is operated by a computer, similar to tossing a coin, to determine who will receive the treatment being tested. A group of patients who agree to help test the new treatment are assigned to receive either the new, unestablished treatment (if the "coin" lands heads-up) or an apparently identical inert treatment called a placebo (if the "coin" lands tails-up). Alternatively, if there is already an established treatment, the new treatment will be compared with this. The enormous advantage of random allocation is that it produces two virtually identical groups of patients. We then can be confident at the end of the study that any differences that appear during the study must be due to the different treatments. If the group that received the new drug does better (has fewer symptoms, feels healthier, lives longer), we can be confident that the drug does more good than harm and is better than the placebo or alternative treat-

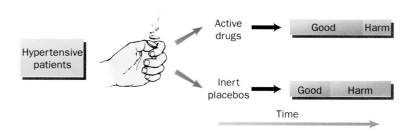

Figure 3-1: Design of a randomized clinical trial

ment to which it was compared. When this happens, we can make this treatment available to similar patients everywhere.

If, on the other hand, both groups look and feel the same at the end of the trial, then we know that the drug is either not more effective than the placebo or alternative treatment to which it is being compared, or that whatever good it may do is balanced by some bad side-effects. When this result occurs, we know that we have to keep looking for a better treatment. Finally, we sometimes find the group receiving the active drug actually does worse than the group receiving placebos! When this happens, we must warn other clinicians and patients not to use this treatment for that condition.

Double-Blind Randomized Trials

In randomized trials that involve the testing of drugs, the active and placebo pills are made to look, feel, smell and taste the same. Moreover, in most randomized trials, both the patient and the patient's physician have agreed not to be told whether the patient is receiving the treatment that is being tested or the placebo or comparison treatment. Thus, their conclusions about the drug's effectiveness will not be influenced (or "biased") by knowing which treatment was being received. When both the patient and the physician are "blind" to which treatment the patient is receiving, the study is called a "double-blind" trial.

What Have We Learned from Randomized Trials?

Randomized clinical trials have proven that several treatments really do more good than harm. Examples of such treatments are the polio vaccine, the coronary bypass operation, and good old aspirin for "little strokes". The results are impressive. Poliomyelitis is now a very rare disease. Thousands of people who would once have been crippled by heart disease are now leading normal lives. Men with little strokes who take aspirin are now only half as likely to suffer or die from big strokes.

Randomized clinical trials have also proven that certain treatments are worthless or even harmful. One example is the "gastric freeze" for peptic ulcer, a treatment in which super-cooled fluid was circulated through the stomach in an effort to stop the production of stomach acid. Another example is big doses of vitamin C for cancer. A third is a bypass operation in which an artery from the scalp is attached to an artery supplying the brain to prevent strokes. The result of these important studies is that patients are no longer subjected to these useless treatments. The money, time and effort previously wasted on them can now be put to better use.

Randomized Trials in Hypertension

Some of the first randomized clinical trials ever conducted were carried out to test whether the treatment of high blood pressure did more good than harm. They began with very severe hypertension. In the 1960s, 143 men with diastolic blood pressures (diastolic being the lower of the two blood pressure readings, representing the pressure in the large arteries between heartbeats) of between 115 and 129 mm Hg agreed to join this first trial. Seventy were randomly assigned to receive inert pills (placebos). The other 73 were randomly assigned to receive active pills containing drugs that would lower their blood pressure.

During the months that followed, 27 of the 70 men taking the inert placebos (that is, 39% of them) suffered complications of their hypertension, such as strokes, severe damage to their eyes, hearts or kidneys, or even death. Over this same time, however, the 73 men taking the active drugs fared much better. Only two of these 73 men (or 3% of them) suffered complications of their hypertension.

It quickly became plain to the doctors in charge of this trial that the men receiving the active pills were faring well, while the men receiving placebos were suffering strokes, heart failure, failure of their eyes and kidneys, and even death. They acted quickly. As soon as it became clear that this dramatic difference could not be due to chance, the trial was stopped, and the men who had been taking the placebos were started on active medicine. We had clear proof, for the first time, that treating high blood pressure did more good than harm.

Recent Trials in Hypertension

The trial involving patients with very severe hypertension was only the beginning of the story. What about less severe elevations in blood pressure? More randomized clinical trials followed. In each of them patients with successively less severe elevations in blood pressure agreed to be randomized to inert placebos or active drugs. Every time, the answer was the same: treating high blood pressure does more good than harm.

However, as patients with less and less severe hypertension joined these studies, two additional answers became clear. First, as suggested from earlier community studies (such as the famous Framingham Heart Epidemiology Study), the smaller the elevation in blood pressure, the smaller the increase in the risk of hypertensive complications. Second, more and more patients with milder hypertension had to be treated for every complication prevented through active treatment.

For example, the earliest trials among the most severely hypertensive patients showed us that, without treatment, two of every three would have a disabling stroke or die within 5 years. With treatment, we could prevent half of these serious complications. Thus, we need to treat just three such persons for 5 years to prevent one of them from dying or having a disabling stroke.

With mild hypertension the risk of such serious complications is much less. Without treatment, only four of every 200 mild hypertensives suffer a disabling stroke or die within 5 years. With treatment, we could prevent a quarter of these serious complications, so we need to treat 200 such persons for 5 years to prevent one of them from dying or having a disabling stroke.

Unfortunately, we cannot tell beforehand which four of these 200 people are the ones destined for stroke or death. We also don't know ahead of time which of these four will be the one who benefits from treatment. Therefore, we must ask all 200 of them to take the treatment. Of course, this also means they must spend the money for the medicine and run the risks, though small, of side-effects from the antihypertensive drugs.

It should come as no surprise to you to learn there is vigorous debate among the "experts" about whether these mildest hypertensive patients should be treated at all, and especially with drugs. Some of this debate dissipates when a person's other risk factors for cardiovascular disease are taken into account. Thus, for two people with the same, mildly high blood pressure without complications, treatment is more likely to be prescribed for the one who has such risk factors as being male, being diabetic, having high blood cholesterol, or having a strong family history for cardiovascular disease.

Whatever disagreement there might be about the need for treatment among people with mild hypertension, there is unanimity about the more severe forms of hypertension. We all agree that anyone with a diastolic blood pressure of 100 mm Hg or more will benefit from treatment, even when they are well along in years. In addition, even individuals with smaller elevations (between 90 and 100), who also show some evidence that the high blood pressure has affected their hearts, brains, eyes or kidneys, have been proven to benefit from treatment.

Moreover, randomized trials have now shown that elderly people with hypertension clearly benefit from treatment, even if just their systolic blood pressure reading is elevated.

The Search Goes On

As you read this book, we are beginning to find that individuals whose diabetes has affected their kidneys benefit from certain types of antihypertensive drugs, even when their blood pressures are normal without treatment. We are also beginning to learn more about which blood pressure-lowering drugs are preferred by patients. Research on this important topic is intense at present, aided by our ability to measure the "quality of life" of patients. New drugs are being developed all the time as well, providing more options for treatment and the promise of fewer adverse effects. We will know much more in the next few years.

Many patients with high blood pressure, and many of us who treat them, would prefer to use special diets (low in salt), weight reduction, special methods of relaxation, or physical exercise if these alternatives to drugs could effectively lower blood pressure and prevent the complications of hypertension. Accordingly, recent randomized trials have considered several of these non-drug treatments of hypertension. You will read about their results in the next two chapters in this book.

Conclusion

Let us end where we began: Why treat high blood pressure? Treating high blood pressure can prevent or reverse most complications of high blood pressure. We have learned that treating high blood pressure does more good than harm by applying rigorous scientific methods, most notably the randomized clinical trial, to the study of this treatment. Time and time again, these randomized trials have proven that people with high blood pressure live longer and healthier lives when their hypertension is detected, diagnosed and treated.

These studies are continuing to be carried out. They will continue to provide important answers that will help us improve the treatment of high blood pressure. This research, which will benefit us all, deserves all our support.

HEALTHY EATING AND BLOOD PRESSURE

Darlene Abbott, RN, MSc, Beverley Whitmore, RD, and Arun Chockalingham, PhD

The goal of this chapter is to discuss recommendations for healthy eating that can help to control high blood pressure and reduce cardiovascular risk. The Canadian Heart Health Survey (1990) found that over half the people with high blood pressure were either overweight or had an elevated cholesterol level. The combination of high blood pressure and these risk factors greatly increases the risk of developing cardiovascular disease. We all have some room for improvement in our diets; here is some practical advice on how to eat better. Readers are referred to Chapter 5 for information on other lifestyle factors including alcohol, exercise, stress and smoking.

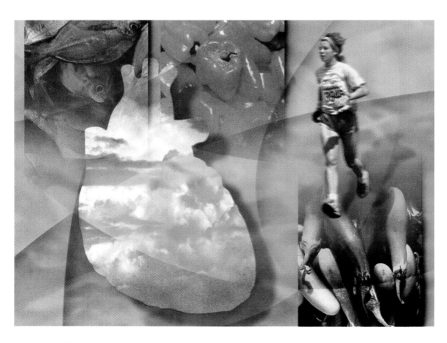

Guide to Healthy Eating

Canada's Food Guide to Healthy Eating is considered an excellent resource on which to pattern your eating habits and is based on the following five principles:

1. A variety of food choices,
2. An increased emphasis on cereals, breads and other grain products, vegetables and fruit,
3. Choices that include lower-fat dairy products, leaner meats, and foods prepared with little or no fat,
4. A healthy body weight that is achieved through a combination of healthy eating and regular exercise, and
5. Limited salt, alcohol and caffeine.

Canada's Food Guide (Fig. 4-1) suggests 1800 to 2400 calories (7560 to 10,080 kilojoules) per day. The number of servings needed daily from the four food groups varies depending on your age, body size, activity and gender. Other foods and beverages that are not part of any food group can be used for flavouring or meal preparation. Some of these foods include fats and oils; jams and sugars; high fat and high salt snacks; water, tea, coffee and soft drinks; and spices and condiments.

This eating style fits well with the eating guidelines for someone with high blood pressure. Look at the *Food Guide* carefully and consider how your present eating style compares to it. Healthy eating doesn't have to cost more either. Choosing foods in season and shopping for sale items will help you stay within your budget.

Obesity and High Blood Pressure

Being overweight is a risk factor in the development of heart disease. Weight loss has also been found to reduce blood pressure in people who have high blood pressure. This effect is

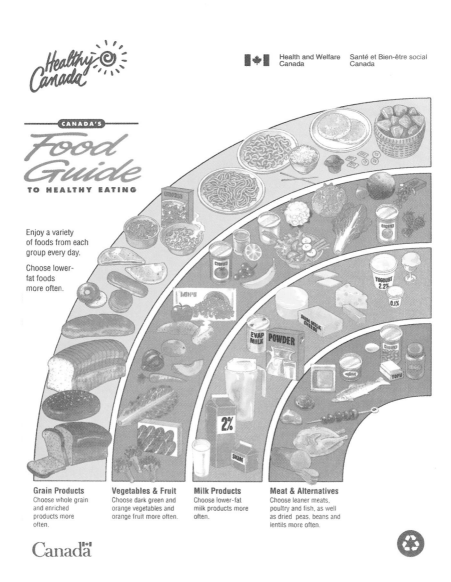

Enjoy a variety
of foods from each
group every day.

Choose lower-
fat foods
more often.

Grain Products
Choose whole grain
and enriched
products more
often.

Vegetables & Fruit
Choose dark green and
orange vegetables and
orange fruit more often.

Milk Products
Choose lower-fat
milk products more
often.

Meat & Alternatives
Choose leaner meats,
poultry and fish, as well
as dried peas, beans and
lentils more often.

Figure 4-1: Canada's Food Guide to Healthy Eating

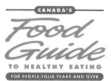

CANADA'S

Food Guide

TO HEALTHY EATING

FOR PEOPLE FOUR YEARS AND OVER

Different People Need Different Amounts of Food

The amount of food you need every day from the 4 food groups and other foods depends on your age, body size, activity level, whether you are male or female and if you are pregnant or breast-feeding. That's why the Food Guide gives a lower and higher number of servings for each food group. For example, young children can choose the lower number of servings, while male teenagers can go to the higher number. Most other people can choose servings somewhere in between.

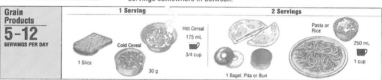

Grain Products
5-12
SERVINGS PER DAY

1 Serving — 1 Slice; Cold Cereal 30 g; Hot Cereal 175 mL 3/4 cup

2 Servings — 1 Bagel, Pita or Bun; Pasta or Rice 250 mL 1 cup

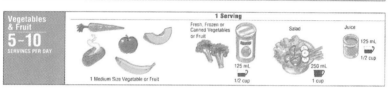

Vegetables & Fruit
5-10
SERVINGS PER DAY

1 Serving — 1 Medium Size Vegetable or Fruit; Fresh, Frozen or Canned Vegetables or Fruit 125 mL 1/2 cup; Salad 250 mL 1 cup; Juice 125 mL 1/2 cup

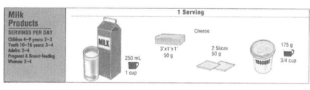

Milk Products
SERVINGS PER DAY
Children 4–9 years: 2–3
Youth 10–16 years: 3–4
Adults: 2–4
Pregnant & Breast-feeding Women: 3–4

1 Serving — 250 mL 1 cup; Cheese 3"x1"x1" 50 g; 2 Slices 50 g; 175 g 3/4 cup

Other Foods

Taste and enjoyment can also come from other foods and beverages that are not part of the 4 food groups. Some of these foods are higher in fat or Calories, so use these foods in moderation.

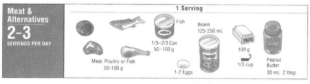

Meat & Alternatives
2-3
SERVINGS PER DAY

1 Serving — Meat, Poultry or Fish 50–100 g; Fish 1/3–2/3 Can 50–100 g; 1-2 Eggs; Beans 125–250 mL 100 g 1/3 cup; Peanut Butter 30 mL 2 tbsp

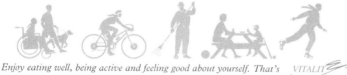

Enjoy eating well, being active and feeling good about yourself. That's VITALIT

© Minister of Supply and Services Canada 1992 Cat. No. H39-252/1992E No changes permitted. Reprint permission not required.
ISBN 0-662-19648-1

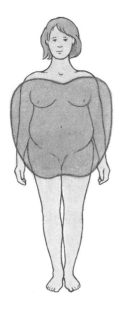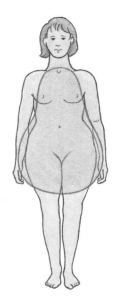

Figure 4-2: Fat concentration and body shape

more dramatic in those who are obese, and a reduction of blood pressure can occur with a weight loss of as little as 10 pounds (4.5 kg). It is important to note, however, that weight loss may not result in blood pressure lowering for some people, just as being overweight does not always mean that the blood pressure will be elevated. Thus, you and your doctor will need to monitor your blood pressure as you lose weight.

There is also evidence that some overweight people are at greater risk than others. Recent research has shown that people who have their fat concentrated in the waist and abdomen (the "apple" shape) are more likely to develop high blood pressure than if the excess fat is located on the thigh or buttocks (the "pear" shape) (Fig.4-2). The measure of distribution of body fat is referred to as a waist-to-hip ratio (WHR).

You can calculate your WHR by dividing your waist circumference by your hip circumference. To measure your waist, place the measuring tape at the point of waist narrowing,

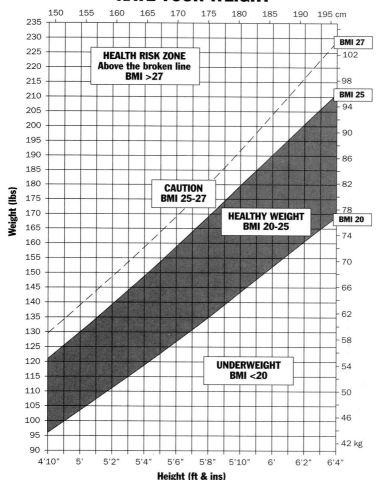

RATE YOUR WEIGHT

Figure 4-3: Rate your Weight — select your height (feet/inches across the bottom, centimetres across the top). Follow its vertical line until it crosses the horizontal line of your body weight (pounds on the left side, kilograms on the right). If your height and weight cross in the stippled area, you are in the healthy body weight range, BMI 20-25. If your height and weight cross above the dotted line, you are in the CAUTION RANGE, BMI 25-27. Any further weight gain is not recommended. If your height and weight cross above the broken line, with a BMI greater than 27, you are too heavy, and you should consider losing some weight. If they cross below the stippled area, with a BMI less than 20, you are thin and should not strive to lose more weight. (Reprinted with the permission of the Health Department, Regional Municipality of Ottawa-Carlton, Ottawa, Ontario.)

breathe out and measure to the nearest centimetre. For the hips, use the measurement of the largest bulge below the waist. Record the measurement as in the following example:

$$\text{WHR} = \frac{\text{waist measurement}}{\text{hip measurement}} = \frac{96 \text{ centimetres}}{102 \text{ centimetres}} = 0.94$$

Values greater than 0.9 in males and 0.8 in females are associated with an increased risk of hypertension and cardiovascular disease. The risk can be decreased by losing weight.

Before we tell you how to lose weight sensibly, it might be helpful for you to know the healthy weight range for you. The *Canadian Guidelines* recommend that all adults aim for a body mass index (BMI★) of 20 to 27, and that all overweight persons being treated for hypertension reduce their weight. The BMI combines both height and weight to assess a person's level of fatness and includes weight from all body sources. You can determine your BMI by using the nomogram (Fig. 4-3). Please note that this index applies only to adults 20 to 65 years of age and does not make allowances for increased muscle mass (for example, in athletes) or distribution of body fat. Thus, this is only a guideline. You and your doctor or nutritionist should discuss what weight is healthiest for you. Even if you are not overweight, much of the advice below will still be of value for keeping you healthy.

Sensible Weight Control

Forget everything you have heard or read about quick weight loss schemes. There are no easy shortcuts. Sensible weight control can only be achieved with consistent healthy eating habits and regular exercise. Maintaining these lifestyle changes will

★ BMI is an estimate of body fatness and is equal to weight in kilograms divided by height in metres squared (kg/m^2)

offer you the greatest chance of success. The following points will help you direct your weight loss efforts.

1. Set a realistic goal weight — start with a weight loss goal of a few pounds during a specified period of time, for example, lose 4 pounds over a month (1 pound a week), then reassess.

2. Participate in some form of regular exercise at least 30 minutes at a time, at least three to four times a week. This doesn't have to be intense or strenuous exercise, but you do have to move your large muscles, especially the legs. For example, a regular walking program has helped many people achieve and maintain weight loss. Think of ways you can increase your activity in your daily routines. Take the stairs instead of the elevator and use a hand-pushed lawn mower instead of a motorized model. Any kind of exercise can help you lose weight. For more details, see Chapter 5.

3. Eat less fat. Switch to skimmed or partially skimmed milk and decrease your intake of butter, margarine, salad dressing and mayonnaise. Trim the fat from meats and the skin from poultry. Other examples of decreasing fat are:

• choose two slices of bread for your sandwich instead of a croissant and

• choose one half cup of skim milk yogurt instead of ice cream. Each of these suggestions will save you 100 calories, all from fat.

4. Eat regular meals. Skipping meals can lead to binge eating and make it harder for you to maintain any weight loss.

5. Increase the fibre content in your diet. Fibre helps to keep you from feeling hungry between meals. Whole grain products, fruits, vegetables, and legumes are high fibre sources.

6. Eat in moderation. Traditional dieting involving severe calorie restriction rarely works for the long term. As hunger is a strong physiologic desire, the body responds to caloric restriction as if starvation were at hand. The eventual result is binge eating and the potential for greater fat storage. Choosing healthy foods and eating just until satisfied will enable you to lose weight more successfully than severely restricting your calories.

7. Moderate your intake of sugar, sweets and alcohol (see Chapter 5).

A safe weight loss is considered to be in the range of 1 to 2 pounds (1/2 to 1 kg) a week. You can ask your doctor to refer you to a dietitian to get more information on healthy eating, label reading and meal preparation. You may also need some professional advice on an exercise program.

Salt and High Blood Pressure

For some time now, it has been thought that salt plays an important role in the development of high blood pressure.[†] Evidence to support this theory comes mostly from studying different populations of the world. The results have shown that primitive societies have a low sodium intake and a low incidence of high blood pressure. Western societies, however, have a high intake of sodium and have higher rates of hypertension. What is not so clear, however, is whether a high salt intake causes hypertension or whether other lifestyle factors (such as exercise or alcohol intake) are involved.

The INTERSALT study, involving 32 countries, was undertaken to settle, once and for all, whether salt is related to blood pressure.

The results did show that blood pressure goes up as salt intake increases. However, the overall effect was quite small, particularly on the diastolic pressure. What seemed to be more closely related to lower blood pressure was the dietary combination of a lower salt and higher potassium intake. As a low

[†] Salt and "sodium" are used interchangeably throughout this chapter. Table salt is made up of two elements, sodium and chloride, and is often referred to as "sodium chloride".

salt, high potassium diet tends to include mostly fresh foods, it may have an added benefit of helping with weight loss through decreased calorie intake. The researchers concluded that the dietary changes that are normally found on a low salt diet could potentially result in a drop of blood pressure averaging 2 to 3 mm Hg. Even this small drop in blood pressure could have a positive effect on the general population and reduce the overall incidence of high blood pressure. However, it is important to point out that the INTERSALT study did not actually test whether lowering salt intake would lower pressure. Studies that have done this have shown little or no effects unless the salt intake is reduced to less than half that in the usual North American diet.

Sodium restriction can reduce blood pressure in some people with high blood pressure and has also been found to enhance the effect of most drugs used in the treatment of high blood pressure (with the exception of calcium antagonists — see Chapter 10). Reducing salt intake could reduce the amount of medication required to control blood pressure. But don't alter the medication on your own! You and your doctor will need to work closely to make the necessary adjustments.

Not all people are sensitive to sodium. However, there is no practical way of knowing how a person's blood pressure will respond to a decreased sodium intake. Regardless, it makes good sense for all of us to reduce our salt intake as the amount of sodium in our diet far exceeds our needs.

Most of the salt we eat is hidden. Fifteen percent of our daily sodium intake comes from salt added to food while cooking or eating and about 10% is naturally present in the food we eat. The remaining 75% comes primarily from processed foods and "fast foods". Therefore, reading product labels to determine the amount of sodium already added to the food you eat becomes an important part of food selection. It is recommended that your total daily intake does not exceed 2000 to 2500 milligrams.

Table 4-1: Sodium Content of Some Commonly Used Foods*

Low Sodium	Sodium (mg)	High Sodium	Sodium (mg)
Roast beef sandwich	270	Large cheeseburger	944
		Pizza slice	540
		Plain hot dog with bun	866
Roast chicken (2 slices)	32	Salami – 2 slices	532
Corn on the cob (4")	trace	Canned corn (1/2 c)	210
Frozen corn (1/2 c)	3		
Apple juice (8 oz)	16	Tomato juice	878
Homemade chicken noodle soup (1 c)	10	Canned chicken soup	1107
Plain popcorn (1 c)	1	Potato chips (10)	200
Part skim mozzarella cheese	132	Cheese spread	381
Soup crackers		Soup crackers	
– nonsalted tops (2)	40	– salted tops (2)	136
Lemon juice (1 tbsp)	0	Soya sauce (1 tbsp)	1029
Fresh salsa (unsalted – 1 tbsp)	5	Canned salsa (1 tbsp)	100
Sliced cucumber (5 – 7 slices)	4	Dill pickle (1 large)	1428

*Values may vary with cooking methods or brand names.

Our taste preference for salt is an acquired habit and will greatly diminish after a few months of restricted intake. Set aside 3 to 6 months to slowly decrease your intake. This should be a more tolerable way for you to make permanent changes in your diet. The first step is to avoid adding salt to food served at the table. Once the food tastes acceptable to you, begin to analyze your food purchasing patterns. Choose fresh or frozen foods rather than canned or packaged items. Become familiar with reading food labels. Ingredients are listed in order of the amount used in the product. Nutrition information is given for the product as it is sold. It does not include ingredients added to complete products such as eggs added to a cake mix. The following is a label from frozen chicken nuggets:

"This product contains chicken, *salt*, lemon juice, spices. Bread crumb coating contains modified starch, wheat flour, corn flour, *salt*, hydrogenated vegetable oil, *baking powder*, soy flour, milk solids, dried egg white, spices, guar gum and *monosodium glutamate*."

The point in reading labels is to avoid salt or sodium compounds found in food products (in this example they have been italicized). If these are listed near the beginning of the ingredient list or if there are two or more sodium sources listed, then you should avoid buying it. It would be better to barbecue a fresh chicken breast rather than eating the chicken nuggets. The less processed a food is, the less sodium it will contain. Look at the values on Table 4-1 to confirm this. Decreasing your salt intake will allow you to get used to the taste of natural foods. You may be surprised at how good a fresh tomato tastes without salt! If you want to add flavour to your foods there are a number of herbs and spices you can use. A low salt cookbook will provide you with many ideas, but here are a few suggestions.

Ground beef: chili powder, oregano, allspice, basil, savory, rosemary
Roast chicken: ginger, cinnamon, poultry seasoning, thyme
Potatoes: parsley, chopped green pepper, onion, rosemary (added to water during cooking).

For more suggestions on how to use flavourings, contact your local dietitian or the Heart and Stroke Foundation.

Alcohol

Alcohol and high blood pressure are discussed in Chapter 5 and are reviewed only briefly here. There is convincing evidence that drinking alcohol increases blood pressure. Drinking alcohol can lead to the development of high blood pressure in some individuals and may worsen the blood pressure in those who already have high blood pressure. You should limit your alcohol intake to a maximum of two standard drinks per day. A standard drink is 120 mL (4 oz) of wine, or 30 mL (1 oz) of liquor, or 340 mL (12 oz) of beer.

Potassium

Populations who consume foods high in potassium have lower blood pressures. A diet rich in potassium is, by its very nature, also low in sodium (salt). It is probably the combination of a low sodium and a high potassium diet that is most important in preventing the development of hypertension.

High potassium diets have been found to lower blood pressures in some individuals being treated for hypertension. Some studies have used potassium pills as a way of increasing potassium in the body. These have also been found to reduce blood pressure, although the effect is usually only for a short time. A potassium-rich diet is especially important for people who are taking certain diuretics (water pills) for their high blood pressure because these pills deplete the body potassium.

Increasing the amount of potassium in your diet will not harm you if you have normal kidney function. (*Note*: If you have kidney disease, do not alter your potassium intake without consulting your doctor.) A potassium-rich diet, in combination with a low salt diet, is especially recommended for those individuals being treated with thiazide diuretics.

Contrary to what you may have heard, you do not have to eat 10 bananas a day or drink a gallon of orange juice to get enough potassium! If you follow the *Food Guide*, you will receive the required amount of potassium for good health. If, for some reason, your body cannot maintain an adequate level of potassium (for example, certain diseases and some medica-

Table 4-2: Foods High in Potassium

Excellent Sources of Potassium
(500+ mg/serving)

Good Sources of Potassium
(300–500 mg/serving)

Peas and Beans
1 cup (250 mL) chick peas,
split peas, common white beans,
red kidney beans, soy beans or
lima beans

Nuts and Seeds
1/2 c (125 mL) almonds and
peanuts (shelled), or sunflower
seeds

Vegetables
1 cup (250 mL) beet greens, parsnips,
pumpkin, spinach, winter squash,
tomato or vegetable juice –1 medium
(100 g) potato (baked in skin)

Fruits
1/2 cup (125 mL) seedless raisins
1 cup (250 mL) orange or prune
juice, rhubarb
1/2 medium (142 g) avocado
1/2 medium (385 g) cantaloupe or
honeydew
1 medium (175 g) banana
1 medium (304 g) papaya
1– 4" x 8" slice watermelon (925 g)
5 halves (72 g) dried peaches
10 halves (79 g) dried apricots
10 medium (100 g) dates, pitted

Milk
1 cup (250 mL) whole, 2%, skim,
buttermilk, reconstituted skim
milk (25g powder: 250 mL), or
goat milk

Meat, Liver, Fish
3 oz (90 g) any cut of beef (lean)
and pork (lean) or cod, halibut,
salmon, scallops, sardines

Lentils and Nuts
1 cup (250 mL) lentils
1/2 cup (125 mL) brazil nuts,
cashew nuts or pecans
1 tbsp (15 mL) peanut butter

Vegetables
1 cup (250 mL) beets, broccoli,
brussel sprouts, carrots,
cauliflower, celery, eggplant,
spinach, summer squash,
turnips, tomatoes, zucchini, or
mushrooms
1 medium (100 g) sweet potato or
potato (peeled, boiled)

Fruits
1 cup (250 mL) grapefruit,
pineapple or tangerine juice or
apricot nectar
1/2 medium (241 g) grapefruit
1 medium (150 g) orange

Adapted from: Foods High in Potassium, Calgary Health Services,
Nutrition Division.

tions can cause you to lose potassium), you may have to increase the amount of potassium-rich foods you eat. Check with your doctor to find out what is best for you.

As well as eating foods from all four food groups, potassium intake can be increased by preparing foods in certain ways. Cooking in a lot of water has the effect of removing potassium. This can be prevented by cooking in a small amount of water and by leaving the skins on vegetables, cutting food into large pieces when boiling, and cooking until just tender. Save the cooking water to use in soups or stews. Try steaming or baking your vegetables, or use a microwave oven. Examples of foods that are high in potassium are listed in Table 4-2. They have been divided into two categories — excellent and good sources of potassium.

Calcium

There is some evidence to suggest that a low calcium intake is associated with an increased rate of high blood pressure. Although a slight decrease in blood pressure has been noted with an increased calcium intake, the results are inconclusive. For now, the best advice is to maintain an adequate intake of calcium. Adequate calcium intake may be helpful in preventing other conditions, such as osteoporosis.

Cholesterol

Do you know what your cholesterol level is? Although the level does not directly affect your blood pressure, high blood cholesterol increases the chances of developing heart disease. The Heart Health Survey found that over half the people with high blood pressure also had an elevated blood cholesterol. The combination of these major risk factors increases the risk of heart disease five-fold. So controlling your cholesterol level should also be one of your goals. Here are some guidelines to help you.

1. Reduce your total fat intake. Avoid high fat foods, frying or deep frying. Limit the use of oil, margarine, butter, salad dressings, gravy and sauces. Limit fat hidden in baked products, fast foods and casseroles.

2. Reduce intake of saturated fats from animal products such as meat, butter, lard, homogenized milk and cheese.

3. Use moderate amounts of polyunsaturated fats such as corn oil, safflower or soybean oils and monounsaturated fats like canola, olive or peanut oil.

4. Limit high cholesterol foods including meats, organ meats, high fat dairy products, egg yolks, butter and shrimp.

5. Achieve a healthy body weight.

6. Exercise regularly.

7. Increase fibre intake, especially foods high in soluble fibre such as dried peas, beans or lentils, fruits and vegetables, and whole grain products.

8. Limit intake of sugar and alcohol.

Menu Planning and Restaurant Meals

Time is precious, which adds to the challenge of meal preparation. The result is an increasing consumption of "convenience" foods from both the grocery store and from fast-food restaurants. These meals tend to be high in salt, fat and calories and may not be suitable for someone who has high blood pressure. If you find that you are eating convenience foods often, ask yourself some questions. Do you enjoy these meals? Are they really saving you time? Have you ever stopped to calculate the cost of these "convenience" meals? Is this a healthy diet? If you answered NO to any of these questions, you probably need to make some changes in your eating habits.

First, do some menu planning (for a week at a time). This may only take 15 minutes of your time. It doesn't have to be detailed. Plan meals that are simple and quick to prepare. Then, make a grocery list from your menu so you can have all the ingredients on hand. Finally, all members of the family should be involved in meal preparation. Children will often eat better when they have helped prepare a meal.

The following are a few quick dinner ideas:

1. Marinated flank steak, sliced on a wholewheat bun served with slices of tomato and onion.
2. Chicken or beef and vegetable stir fry with rice or noodles.
3. Diced cooked chicken and vegetables in a yogurt sauce wrapped in a tortilla or crepe.
4. Hearty beef and vegetable stew simmered all day in a crock pot, served with wholewheat buns.
5. Microwaved fish, baked potato with yogurt and dillweed, mixed vegetable salad with rice vinegar as dressing.
6. Quesidillas — flour tortilla folded over refried beans, diced tomato, salsa, mozzarella cheese and baked.
Add extra vegetables and fruit and a glass of milk to complete the meal.

If you're eating out, these tips will help you enjoy a healthy restaurant meal.

1. Consider what the menu may offer when choosing a restaurant (for example, a fish n' chips restaurant will offer few low fat options).
2. Avoid buffets (people tend to overeat).
3. Eat slowly until you are comfortably full (you don't have to eat everything on your plate).

4. Select foods without cream sauces, gravies, etc. A broiled steak or baked fish with a lemon wedge would be a good choice.

5. Choose food that has been prepared by broiling, steaming, poaching.

6. Enjoy aspects of the meal *other than* food, including the atmosphere, the company and the relaxation associated with eating out.

Conclusions

Diet and lifestyle factors play an important part in the prevention and control of high blood pressure. Reduction of alcohol intake and weight loss (in combination with increased physical activity) are considered to be effective ways of lowering blood pressure. While the effect of salt restriction and increased potassium on blood pressure may be small, reducing salt intake also enhances the effect of most drugs used in the treatment of high blood pressure.

Eating the right kinds of foods is not difficult. Many of the dietary factors discussed tend to be linked together. For example, a high potassium diet will tend to be low in salt and low in cholesterol. Similarly, a restricted calorie diet may be lower in salt. These natural combinations make it easier to make healthy food choices.

By adopting and maintaining healthy eating habits you can help to control your blood pressure and also reduce your risk of heart disease.

Enjoy healthy eating!

LIFESTYLE AND HIGH BLOOD PRESSURE

Jane Irvine, D Phil, and

Jean Cléroux, PhD

Our lifestyle, how we eat, drink, exercise and handle stress, influences our blood pressure, increasing the risk for hypertension and aggravating hypertension once it develops. When we improve these lifestyle factors, blood pressure may be lowered.

Diet and weight are perhaps the most important influences and have already been discussed in Chapter 4. In this chapter, we will first describe the ways alcohol, stress and exercise are related to your blood pressure. We will then discuss the prospects for lowering your blood pressure through improving these aspects of your lifestyle.

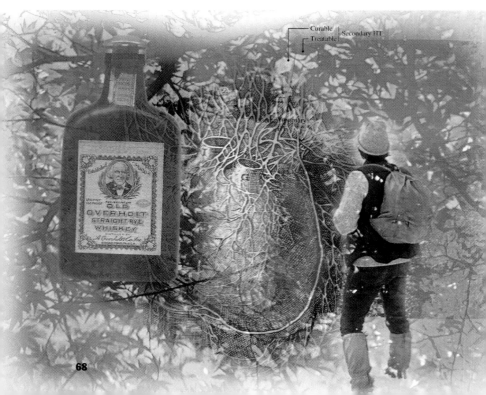

Does Alcohol Raise Blood Pressure ?

Numerous studies have shown that the more alcohol that is consumed the higher the blood pressure and the more likely the development of hypertension. Some reports suggest that the effect of alcohol begins with very small amounts. Thus, people who do not drink alcohol have the lowest blood pressures. Other reports show, however, that there is a threshold at which alcohol consumption affects blood pressure. Thus, one or two alcoholic drinks a day are associated with the same low blood pressures as no drinks, but three or more drinks a day are associated with progressively higher blood pressures. Finally, there are few studies which report that individuals who drink one or two alcoholic drinks a day have lower blood pressures than either those who abstain or those who drink more than the equivalent of three alcoholic drinks a day. In other words, taking three or four drinks per day is certainly harmful, but it is unclear whether consumption below this level affects blood pressure.

It is also of interest that one or two drinks per day raises the amount of "high-density lipoprotein". This, in turn, *lowers* the amount of fatty cholesterol that clogs your arteries (atherosclerosis). Thus, from the perspective of hypertension and atherosclerosis at least, one to two alcoholic drinks per day actually may be beneficial.

By the way, there is no proof that one type of alcoholic beverage is better for your blood pressure than another. What matters is the total amount of alcohol consumed. Furthermore, common sense dictates that even the consumption of one or two drinks a day could be dangerous before driving a vehicle, operating potentially dangerous machinery, or in other situations requiring sharp wits and reflexes.

Does Cigarette Smoking Raise Blood Pressure ?

Cigarette smoking is not a cause of hypertension. It does, however, cause a temporary increase in blood pressure by about 10 mm Hg systolic pressure and 8 mm Hg diastolic pressure while smoking and shortly thereafter. Of even more importance to the hypertensive patient, cigarette smoking appears to cancel the beneficial effects of some antihypertensive medications. For example, one large hypertension treatment trial found that beta-blocker therapy (see Chapter 8) decreased the risk of heart disease and stroke *only among those who did not smoke.* Furthermore, cigarette smoking is one of the most important risk factors for coronary heart disease, stroke and cancer. Risk factors potentiate one another. If you both smoke and have hypertension you are at much greater risk of heart disease and stroke than if you had only one of these risk factors.

Does Acute Stress Raise Blood Pressure ?

There is a well-known response of the body to acute stress, termed the alarm reaction, the defense reaction or the "fight or flight" response. This is characterized by an increase in blood pressure, heart rate, respiratory rate and muscle tension. There is also an increase in blood flow to the skeletal muscles and decrease in blood flow to the skin, kidneys and bowels. As discussed in Chapter 1, these responses are activated via the autonomic nervous system. Hormones such as adrenaline and noradrenaline are released into the blood and further stimulate the body. This response is natural and healthy and helps the body to respond to danger. However, this response to stressors may be inappropriate when it occurs where no course of action is possible. In other words, if this alarm response is not followed by some course of action such as fight or flight, then the body is aroused beyond what is required.

The alarm response is usually short-lived, decreasing rapidly when the stress is over. However, it may be harmful in individuals who have either a family history for hypertension or an existing cardiovascular disease. This is because in these individuals the increase in blood pressure tends to be greater and more prolonged.

Is Chronic Stress Associated with Hypertension ?

In some situations, a chronic state of alarm has been associated with high blood pressure. For example, hypertension was found to be more common among people exposed to combat during World War II and among men anticipating unemployment when their place of work was to be shut down. Therefore, certain stressful conditions can produce a sustained elevation in blood pressure. However, in these studies, blood pressure was found to return to normal once conditions returned to normal.

Perhaps if the stressful conditions were more prolonged, the increase in blood pressure would become permanent. This possibility has been tested by researchers who studied people exposed to long-term stressful conditions. These studies found a higher likelihood of hypertension in certain jobs such as air traffic control and among manual or machine workers who reported that their superiors were generally unsupportive. Working or living in very noisy conditions also has been linked with higher rates of hypertension.

High blood pressure has also been found to be more common in people who reside in high stress neighbourhoods where crime rates, marital break-up rates, the number of residents and resident instability were high, and income was low. Researchers have been trying to understand what it is about these kinds of conditions that raise blood pressure. It has been suggested that a common feature of these situations is that people have too many demands and too little personal control over these demands. Thus, where demands are high and personal control low there may be a chronic state of stress.

These studies provide some evidence that chronic stress is related to hypertension, but they do not explain why. Is this explained by the acute stress reaction with the associated increase in adrenaline or noradrenaline? Or do other risk factors account for the relationship between stress and hypertension, such as high rates of alcohol consumption due to stress? As yet, we do not have answers to these questions.

Just the same, most people exposed to stress do not develop hypertension. This finding has led to the theory that individuals may differ in their sensitivity to the blood pressure effects of stress.

Characteristics That May Make People More Sensitive to Stress

Both genetic factors and personality factors have been studied to see if these explain why only some people develop hypertension when under stress. There is good evidence that a positive family history for hypertension makes the individual prone to react with exaggerated increases in blood pressure when stressed. However, we do not know yet if this exaggerated blood pressure reaction leads to a permanent increase in blood pressure.

The results to date on personality factors, such as anxious or angry personality styles, indicate that these characteristics are not linked with developing hypertension. Rather, increased anxiety and anger are common in diagnosed hypertensive individuals and so may be a result of knowledge of hypertension, not its cause. Studies of individuals who are not aware that they have hypertension have found that these unaware hypertensives are no more anxious or angry than individuals who have normal levels of blood pressure.

Does Hypertension Cause Stress?

This is an important question because many people with hypertension who feel that they are under stress may in fact be reacting to the discovery of their hypertension.

Learning about one's hypertension, that is, *hypertension labelling*, has been associated with many adverse consequences. Some of these consequences include decreased time spent in social/leisure activities, increased work absenteeism, decreased financial earnings, increased anxiety and anger, worry about health, and physical symptoms such as headaches. Health professionals are becoming increasingly aware of these adverse psychological effects. They are making an effort to help patients understand hypertension better to reduce worry.

The best method to reduce the effects of hypertension labelling appears to be effective blood pressure treatment. For example, patients whose blood pressures are well controlled by medication appear to suffer fewer of these adverse consequences. If you recognize some of these problems in yourself, then it might be helpful to understand that these may be due to your concern or worry about your blood pressure and not due to the high blood pressure itself. Overcoming these problems begins with the recognition that effective treatment eliminates almost all of the health risk due to hypertension. If your blood pressure is well controlled, you can lead a normal life in almost every way. Be sure to raise any concerns you may have with your doctor so he or she can help you.

Does Lack of Regular Physical Exercise Affect Blood Pressure?

The first indirect evidence of a relationship between the level of physical activity and the later development of hypertension came from two studies performed in the late 1960s and 1970s by Dr. R. S. Paffenbarger and his colleagues in the United

States. These researchers found that the incidence of hypertension was 20% to 40% lower in those who had participated in at least 5 hours of sports activities per week during their college years than in people who were less active in their younger years. Moreover, those individuals who had slower heart rates when in college (physical training slows the heart rate at rest) were also less likely to have hypertension 20 to 30 years later. This finding, together with a report that slowing the heart rate (in animals) can retard atherosclerosis (clogging of the arteries), suggests that physical training may exert a preventive action in more than one way. This view is supported by the results of a study published in 1986 by the same group of investigators. This showed that active people live longer even when high blood pressure, smoking and obesity are taken into account. In 1993, it was shown that initially sedentary men who started to participate in sports activities of moderate intensity had a 40% reduction in the risk of death from coronary heart disease; this was comparable to the reduction in men who stopped smoking.

In other studies, the heart function of hypertensive individuals was examined during physical exercise. These studies showed that abnormalities of the heart occurred less often in people who were physically active than in those who were sedentary.

These findings are encouraging because they indicate that being physically active may lessen the chance of becoming hypertensive or of having an abnormal reaction during exercise if one is already hypertensive. However, they do not show that becoming more physically active can reverse the changes. To determine if physical training can be of any value in the treatment of hypertension, a group of previously inactive hypertensive individuals must undertake an exercise program and its effects on the blood pressure levels examined. Many such studies have been done and show that regular dynamic exercise training can reduce blood pressure by roughly 10 mm Hg in

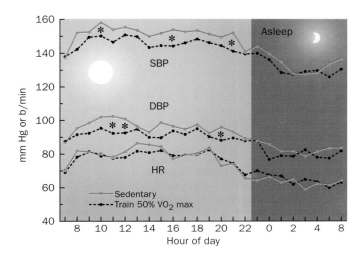

Figure 5-1: Hourly systolic (SBP) and diastolic (DBP) blood pressure and heart rate (HR) of the subjects over 24 hours after the sedentary period and after training at 50% of maximal oxygen uptake (TRAIN 50% VO$_2$ MAX). *Difference is statistically significantly better than sedentary at indicated time points. Note the effect of this training intensity on the morning rise of DBP. (Reproduced, with permission, from Marceau M, Kouamé N, Lacourcière Y, Cléroux J. Effects of different training intensities on 24-hour blood pressure in hypertensive subjects. Circulation 1993; 88:2803–2811. Copyright 1993 American Heart Association.)

subjects with essential hypertension. Results from one such study are shown in Figures 5-1 and 5-2.

It is important to distinguish between dynamic and isometric exercise here. Dynamic exercise involves a large number of repetitions of continuous movements that often require only modest muscle contractions, such as walking, jogging, bicycling, aerobic dancing, swimming, and so on. Isometric exercises involve few repetitions of movements typically requiring more intense muscle contractions during weight lifting, such as those performed on muscle-building machines. During both dynamic and isometric exercise blood pressure normally increases. However, it increases much more during isometric than dynamic exercise. The recommendation of the Canadian consensus conference, co-sponsored by the Canadian Hypertension

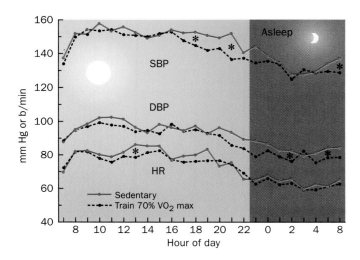

Figure 5-2: Hourly systolic (SBP) and diastolic (DBP) blood pressure and heart rate (HR) of the subjects over 24 hours after the sedentary period and after training at 70% of maximal oxygen uptake (TRAIN 70% VO_2 MAX). *Difference is statistically significantly better than sedentary at indicated time points. Note the absence of effect of this training intensity on blood pressure during work hours (8:00 to 17:00 hours). (Reproduced, with permission, from Marceau M, Kouamé N, Lacourcière Y, Cléroux J. Effects of different training intensities on 24-hour blood pressure in hypertensive subjects. Circulation 1993; 88:2803–2811. Copyright American Heart Association.)

Society, is that activities such as weight lifting are contraindicated. Isometric exercises are thus strongly discouraged, unless performed in closely supervised conditions. (You might want to avoid pushing your car if it is stuck in the snow!)

Blood pressure reduction occurs rapidly during the first weeks of dynamic exercise training with more than 75% of the antihypertensive effect found after 20 weeks already present by 10 weeks. Similarly, more than 75% of the antihypertensive effect that can be obtained by exercising daily is present by exercising every other day. On the other hand, increasing the intensity of exercise does not augment the antihypertensive effect since low- and moderate-intensity training produce similar 24-hour blood pressure reductions. In the study illustrated in Figures 5-1 and 5-2, the low-intensity exercise corresponds to walking at a brisk pace (a mile in 16 minutes), and the moderate intensity training corresponds to jogging at a rate of a mile every 8 minutes. The main difference is that low-intensity training reduces blood pressure to a greater extent during working hours whereas moderate-intensity training has more pronounced antihypertensive effects during the evening and sleep hours (as shown in Figs. 5-1 and 5-2). It was also shown that the antihypertensive effect of the exercise was sustained during a 12-month follow-up period.

It is also important to note that the effect of exercise occurs whether or not there is weight loss. Of course, weight loss has its own effect, and exercise and weight loss complement one another.

Lifestyle Modification

If certain aspects of lifestyle affect blood pressure, then changing these factors may help prevent hypertension or decrease the blood pressure if it is already elevated. Here are some ways to modify alcohol consumption, stress and physical exercise.

Recommendations for Alcohol Consumption

Based on the evidence relating alcohol consumption to blood pressure, the Canadian Hypertension Society has recommended that you should drink no more than two standard alcoholic drinks per day. A standard drink is 120 mL (4 oz) of wine, 30 mL (1 oz) of liquor and 360 mL (12 oz) of beer (Fig. 5-3). The Society also recommends that if the blood pressure is still not controlled, abstinence may be helpful. Also, if you find it difficult to stick to your limit of two standard drinks per day, abstinence may be necessary, at least in the short run to get you started in changing your drinking patterns.

If you drink alcohol, alcohol restriction can be tried as a first step in treating mildly elevated blood pressure, that is, a diastolic blood pressure between 90 and 100 mm Hg. It is also important to note that other types of antihypertensive treatments are likely to be made less effective if you continue to consume excess alcohol. For example, stress management has been shown to be less effective in patients who consume alcohol heavily. The same is likely to apply to antihypertensive medications, diet and exercise.

To begin to change your drinking pattern, it may be helpful to keep a record of (1) the number of abstinent days, moderate drinking days (consumed 1-4 standard drinks), and heavy drinking days (consumed 5 or more drinks) in a month; (2) number of days since last drink; and (3) the duration of this drinking pattern.

Second, alcohol consumption usually fits a pattern that serves a function for you. Some of these functions can involve drinking to (1) reduce negative feelings of tension or sadness; (2) have pleasure; (3) aid some kind of performance (for example, socializing); and (4) reduce social pressure or be part of the crowd. Sometimes drinking can serve no purpose; that is, it

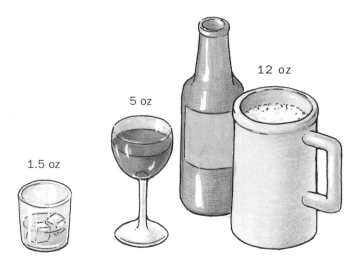

Figure 5-3: Standard drink sizes

is just a habit. Alcohol consumption can have one or more functions in the same individual. Understanding the functions alcohol serves for you can help you find alternatives for each function.

Third, set your own goal. The ultimate goal is to drink no more than two standard drinks per day. At first you may want to set a slightly higher goal of say three drinks if you are used to drinking quite heavily. However, until you reach no more than two drinks per day, you may not experience much of a blood pressure response. In setting a drinking goal, you should specify (1) the maximum number of drinking days per week; (2) the maximum number of drinks on drinking days; (3) when it is okay to drink; (4) when it is not okay to drink (based on your analysis of your drinking pattern); and (5) how long you are going to try to change your drinking pattern (that is, at what point you may want to seek help from an experienced therapist).

Fourth, you may want to try various strategies to help you reach your goal. One strategy is pacing of drinking. Pacing includes measuring each drink, mixing drinks rather than having them straight, sipping drinks rather than gulping them, spacing drinks by alternating alcoholic and nonalcoholic drinks or by letting at least 1 hour pass before taking the next drink, and avoiding drinking on an empty stomach. Another strategy is self-monitoring of drinking. Self-monitoring includes keeping a record of time of alcohol consumption, quantity consumed, function for drinking, urges or temptations to drink, and pressures from others to drink. Self-monitoring will help remind you of your goal, clarify the reasons for your drinking, and identify problem areas.

Fifth, prepare in advance what you will do when alcohol is freely available (remember the pacing tips) or when pressures from others are likely to occur (for example, "Thank you, I'm OK for now."). Set ahead of time the maximum number of drinks you will consume. Be prepared to counteract your own excuses to go over your goal (for example, "I'm not working tomorrow." or "I'm not driving tonight.").

Sixth, take up activities that are incompatible with heavy drinking. For example, take up an educational or physical fitness program, develop or re-activate a hobby, and change your social network to support your drinking goal.

Seventh, problems at home or work may make you feel like drinking. You must set a rule that alcohol should not be used to cope with problems. Find other solutions. You may want to seek help from an experienced therapist for these problems, but often it can help to ask a close friend for advice. If you find that you cannot achieve your drinking goal, then you may find it helpful to ask your doctor to help plan and supervise the program with you. He or she can also refer you to an experienced therapist.

Recommendations about Smoking

It is not easy to quit smoking, but it is particularly important for people with high blood pressure to do so. Many of the tactics discussed for reducing alcohol intake work for cigarette smoking as well. Try them! In addition, there are many helpful aids and programs for quitting smoking these days, including nicotine replacement therapy. If you find it difficult to stop smoking on your own, your doctor can help you or refer you to special clinics or programs.

Recommendations about Relaxation

Relaxation therapy cannot be confidently recommended as a treatment for hypertension. First, it is not certain whether relaxation therapy lowers people's blood pressures over the whole day. Second, there have been no studies to determine if relaxation therapy can prevent hypertensive-related complications such as heart disease and stroke. Thus, the recommendation of the Canadian consensus conference, co-sponsored by the Canadian Hypertension Society, is that it is premature to recommend the use of relaxation/stress management techniques in the treatment of high blood pressure. Nevertheless, some people may experience a fall in blood pressure. Therefore, we recommend that, if you try relaxation therapy or stress management therapy, do so with the agreement and supervision of your doctor so that any effect on your blood pressure can be determined.

Recommendations for Exercise

Physical training may not be beneficial for everyone. If you and your doctor feel that you should increase your exercise, here are some tips on how to get started. First, you must be willing to become more physically active in everyday life. This by no means implies that you should rush off to register for fitness classes right away! Rather, you should begin with more convenient measures; you could get off the bus one stop earlier and walk the remaining distance to your destination. Use the stairways instead of the elevator, or get off the elevator one floor earlier. (We recommend that you start by walking downstairs for a few weeks before walking upstairs. This will impose less of a burden on your heart while improving the strength of your leg muscles).

These are obvious suggestions. You can probably think of many other methods to increase routine exercise. With the tight schedules of life, you may have to make some minor concessions to change your exercise habits. For example, you will find that you have to leave earlier for work if you choose to walk. You may have to take 10 minutes less for lunch if you take the stairs to and from the cafeteria instead of the elevator. If you are not willing to sacrifice the time needed to make these changes, it is unlikely that you will adhere to the demands of a fitness program that involves even more time and expense. On the other hand, if you find that walking for 30 minutes in the evening before supper becomes an enjoyable part of the day, and if you find it rewarding to perform a certain physical task without discomfort, then you probably are the type of person who could benefit further from a carefully supervised exercise program.

At this point, you could start looking for more specialized advice as to the type of exercise you should take up. To begin, seek your doctor's advice once you have told him about your more active lifestyle. He might be able to refer you to an exercise specialist who could assess your general fitness level and recommend an individualized training program for you. If a significant antihypertensive effect of exercise becomes evident, your doctor may want to postpone or modify drug treatment. We emphasize that your doctor must be involved in such decisions. Do not for any reason try to replace medication with an hour of exercise! While such an action may be possible in the long run, persistent blood pressure lowering should be shown before medication is changed. Also, especially if your blood pressure is not well controlled, recall that blood pressure is actually raised during exercise.

Remember that your goal should be a general change in your lifestyle, from sedentary to more active. It is not possible to achieve this overnight! Be patient and persistent! On the positive side, remember that you don't need to become a marathon runner to decrease blood pressure. Walking at a brisk pace may be equivalent to jogging in terms of blood pressure lowering effects.

CHAPTER 6

GENERAL APPROACH
TO TREATMENT OF HYPERTENSION

Martin Myers, MD

In the past 50 years, few advances in medicine surpass the benefits achieved by the development of drugs for the treatment of high blood pressure. Before 1950, there was no practical way to lower blood pressure with or without medications. When a physician made a diagnosis of high blood pressure, it was generally received with great despair since the outcome was often quite dismal. Indeed, patients with the most severe type of high blood pressure had less than a 10% chance of surviving the next 12 months.

Fortunately, medical research and the development of new drugs for the treatment of high blood pressure during the past 40 years have almost completely reversed this gloomy outcome. Between 1950 and 1970, drug treatment of hypertension became increasingly widespread. Most of the attention during this period was directed toward patients with more severe high blood pressure because the drugs often caused troublesome side-effects and were appropriate only for those most likely to benefit. However, by the early 1970s, the availability of drugs called diuretics and beta-blockers made it possible to treat the high blood pressure of most patients effectively with few adverse effects.

Goal of Treatment for High Blood Pressure

We know that lowering blood pressure to less than 140/90 mm Hg will reduce complications. However, there is less certainty about the best blood pressure to aim for. In general, among individuals who are not on treatment, the lower the blood pressure the better off one is. However, with drug treatment there is some evidence that lowering the blood pressure far below 140/90 mm Hg may not give added benefit. Indeed, this may run the risk of more adverse effects. Thus, in most situations, the goal is to lower blood pressure to less than 140/90 mm Hg but not much less than this. The goal differs in the elderly with systolic hypertension (see Chapter 12).

How to Lower Blood Pressure

In patients with mild high blood pressure, the ideal approach is to reduce the blood pressure without using a drug. For example, an obese patient can lose weight, heavy users of alcohol can reduce their intake and everyone can consume less salt (sodium) in the diet. As explained in Chapter 15, it is often difficult for people to follow these instructions. Also, even if adhered to, they may not reduce the blood pressure to the goal of less than 140/90 mm Hg. Thus, for patients with more than just a mild increase in blood pressure and for those who find it difficult to comply with non-drug treatments, blood pressure must be lowered by a medication.

In general, drugs reduce blood pressure by influencing mechanisms that are involved in the normal maintenance of blood pressure, such as the activity of the pump (the heart) and the resistance of the blood vessels to the flow of blood (the arteries through which the heart has to pump blood).

Drugs Currently Available for the Treatment of High Blood Pressure

The medications that are used to treat high blood pressure today have been grouped into five main categories to give an overview. The details of each type of drug are in the chapters that follow.

Diuretics (Water Pills) (Chapter 7)

Diuretics increase the amount of sodium (salt) and water excreted as urine by the kidneys. This action reduces the volume of the blood pumped by the heart with each beat. Diuretics may also decrease the sodium content of blood vessels leading to reduced resistance to flow.

Inhibitors of the Sympathetic Nervous System (Chapter 8)

The brain sends signals along this system that act on the heart and the blood vessels. The sympathetic nervous system works via two hormones (noradrenaline and adrenaline) that stimulate receptors on the walls of some cells of the body. There are two main types of receptors, alpha-receptors and beta-receptors. Stimulation of the alpha-receptors causes constriction of the blood vessels, and stimulation of the beta-receptors causes the heart to pump stronger and faster. Because stimulation of either alpha- or beta-receptors can raise blood pressure, drugs that block alpha- or beta-receptors thus lower the blood pressure. Beta-blockers, therefore, are a subgroup of agents that inhibit part of this system. Other subgroups are alpha-blockers and drugs acting in the brain (centrally acting drugs) to reduce the stimulating effects of the sympathetic nervous system.

Angiotensin Converting Enzyme (ACE) Inhibitors (Chapter 9)

These drugs block the effects of the hormone renin, which is released from the kidney. Renin normally acts to produce other hormones (angiotensins) that constrict arteries. By blocking the actions of renin, converting enzyme inhibitors relax arteries and lower the resistance to blood flow.

Calcium Antagonists (Chapter 10)

These drugs inhibit the entry of calcium into muscle cells in the heart and in the walls of arteries. Because calcium is needed for muscle contraction, these drugs decrease the heart's power

of contraction and output of blood. They also act as vasodilators to reduce the resistance of blood flow in the arteries.

Vasodilators (Chapter 11)
Vasodilators relax the muscle in the walls of arteries. This
action widens these blood vessels and thus decreases the resistance to blood flow.

What Is the Ideal Blood Pressure-Lowering Drug?

The ideal blood pressure-lowering drug would reduce blood
pressure without causing any adverse effects. It would be inexpensive, require infrequent administration, and eliminate all the
complications of high blood pressure. It would also be compat-
ible with other drugs and not affected by other diseases or
medical conditions. As you might expect, we have not yet
achieved perfection. Fortunately we do have a variety of drugs
available that lower blood pressure effectively and have many
other positive attributes.

Recently, the Canadian Hypertension Society convened a
consensus conference to revise existing recommendations on
the drug treatment of high blood pressure. In its deliberations,
the conference used the "ideal" drug as a standard by which to
judge currently available medications. Just about every drug
available for high blood pressure actually lowers the pressure,
but some do it a little better than others. Not all drugs seem to
reduce the complications of high blood pressure, and we may
not have much information on how well a particular drug prevents complications such as stroke and heart disease. This is
especially true if the drug is new. Even though most drugs
cause few important side-effects, some cause fewer than others.

It might seem a simple task to select the drug with the
most favourable characteristics, but unfortunately that is not so.
For example, a new drug may lower blood pressure effectively

and seem to be comparatively free of side-effects. However, a new drug is bound to be more expensive — it costs a great deal to develop and test a new drug. The new drug also will not have been around long enough to know if it has any long-term adverse effects or if it actually reduces the complications of hypertension over a 5- to 10-year period. Thus, an older, less expensive and better known medication has its attractions. Any recommendations on the drug treatment of high blood pressure must consider what we actually know about each drug and what has yet to be discovered, particularly with the newer agents.

Canadian Recommendations for the Treatment of High Blood Pressure with Drugs

Treatment of Patients with Uncomplicated High Blood Pressure (Figure 6-1)

Two types of drugs — diuretics (water pills) or beta-blockers — are recommended as the first choice in treating patients with high blood pressure who do not have complications or other conditions that might influence the selection of appropriate therapy. Lower doses of diuretics are recommended (hydrochlorothiazide 12.5 to 25 mg per day). This is because

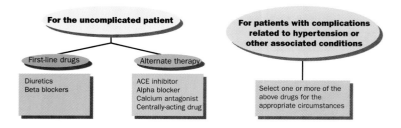

Figure 6-1: General recommendations for drug therapy

we now know that the higher doses used previously were not necessary to lower the blood pressure. At least as important, these higher doses were the main reason many patients experienced adverse effects such as a low potassium in the blood (see Chapter 7 for details).

A beta-blocker or diuretic can be expected to achieve a normal blood pressure in about two thirds of patients with mild or moderate high blood pressure. Sometimes there is only a partial response to the first medication. Rather than adding a second drug at this point, we generally prefer to try the alternate medication. For example, if a beta-blocker has not reduced the blood pressure enough, it could be stopped and replaced with a diuretic or vice versa.

If the blood pressure is not brought down to normal with the diuretic or beta-blocker, there are several options. The beta-blocker and diuretic can be combined using a little of each drug to lower the blood pressure to normal. Alternatively, when the beta-blocker and diuretic have each been tried alone and have failed to normalize the blood pressure, another agent such as an alpha-blocker, ACE inhibitor, calcium antagonist, or centrally acting drug (in alphabetic order) may be prescribed. The aim here is to reduce the blood pressure to normal while still using only one medication. These agents may also be used if the combination of a beta-blocker and diuretic has not achieved an adequate blood pressure response.

Some patients with more severe high blood pressure or those whose blood pressure is somewhat resistant to treatment may require other combinations of drugs. Commonly used combinations include a diuretic and an ACE inhibitor, centrally acting drug or alpha-blocker. Alternatively, a beta-blocker can be given with a vasodilating calcium antagonist or an alpha-blocker. If the use of two drugs does not achieve a normal blood pressure, then three or more agents may be required. Fortunately, this situation arises in less than 10% of patients with high blood pressure.

If there are no complicating factors influencing the choice of therapy, the doctor can follow the general approach outlined above. When the high blood pressure is more difficult to control, it is often necessary to try several different combinations. The goal is to find one or more medications that lower blood pressure adequately with few or no side-effects and at a minimum cost, to find the optimal number of tablets per day, and so on. Just because your doctor does not prescribe the most effective drug or combination of drugs initially does not necessarily mean that he or she is not treating you properly. For reasons that are usually unknown, some patients will respond better to one type of medicine than another. It sometimes takes several attempts before the best drug or combination of drugs is matched to the individual patient.

Having said this, the majority of patients with uncomplicated high blood pressure will achieve an adequate blood pressure response to either a beta-blocker and/or a diuretic.

Treatment of High Blood Pressure in the Presence of Other Disorders

A physician may prefer a particular drug for treating high blood pressure because a patient has another condition that might also benefit from the same medicine. On the other hand, it may not be possible to prescribe certain drugs if a patient has another medical condition that would be adversely affected by the treatment. In order to select the most appropriate blood pressure drug, the doctor assesses the patient for the presence of illnesses such as heart disease, stroke, diabetes, high cholesterol, kidney disease, asthma and gout.

High Blood Pressure and Heart Disease. Patients with high blood pressure and coronary artery disease (who have had a heart attack or suffer from angina) are often prescribed beta-blockers or calcium antagonists. This is because these drugs are beneficial for both the high blood pressure and the heart disease.

Diuretics and ACE inhibitors are often used to treat patients who have a condition called congestive heart failure, which usually involves damage to the heart muscle and an impaired pumping action of the heart. If a patient also has high blood pressure, then a diuretic and/or ACE inhibitor may be used to benefit both conditions. Some drugs may be harmful if heart failure is a major concern. In these instances we would not use a beta-blocker and would generally avoid prescribing a calcium antagonist.

High Blood Pressure and Diabetes. In these individuals, ACE inhibitors are often used to control the high blood pressure and reduce the likelihood that kidney function will decline. Other first-line agents include calcium antagonists and alpha-blockers. As discussed in Chapter 13, diuretics and beta-blockers are less commonly used in patients with both high blood pressure and diabetes.

High Blood Pressure and High Cholesterol. Until recently, there was some concern among doctors treating patients with high blood pressure that diuretics and beta-blockers may cause an increase in cholesterol and other fatty substances (triglycerides) in the body. It is now apparent that the increase in cholesterol previously attributed to diuretics does not occur with the lower dosages that are currently recommended. If cholesterol is a special concern, your doctor may still prescribe a diuretic because this class of drugs is known to reduce morbidity and mortality in patients with hypertension. Alternatively, one of the newer agents that does not adversely affect cholesterol or triglycerides may be used including alpha-blockers, ACE inhibitors, calcium antagonists and centrally acting drugs.

Some beta-blockers do increase the triglyceride content in the body. If this is a concern, then your doctor may decide to prescribe one of the beta-blockers that does not have any effect on either triglycerides or cholesterol.

Asthma. Beta-blockers should not be taken by patients who have had asthma (wheezy breathing not necessarily associated with a respiratory infection). These drugs tend to make breathing more difficult and can make asthma much worse.

Gout. Diuretics can increase the amount of uric acid in the blood. When increased amounts of this substance accumulate in the body, a person may get gout (severe joint inflammation and pain). Gout can usually be treated effectively with other medication. If the diuretic was the cause of the gout (and the patient was not going to develop gout on his/her own anyway), stopping the diuretic will generally abolish further attacks.

High Blood Pressure in Special Circumstances

Pregnant women may develop high blood pressure. Often this responds to bed rest. Sometimes, drug therapy is required. Caution with drug treatment in pregnancy is extremely important and only a few compounds are recommended: methyldopa, hydralazine and beta-blockers. In special circumstances other drugs may be used with care if they are not known to be harmful for the mother or fetus and the blood pressure cannot be controlled otherwise. Further details are provided in Chapter 14.

In the elderly, diuretics are generally preferred over beta-blockers because they seem to be somewhat more effective. We tend to use smaller doses of most drugs in older patients and take special care to avoid inducing any side-effects. More information is given in Chapter 12.

Black patients may respond particularly well to diuretics and so one of these drugs is often prescribed first. Otherwise, treatment is the same as outlined above.

General Approach to Adverse Effects

By far the majority of drugs currently used to treat high blood pressure are well tolerated. However, no drug is totally devoid of adverse effects. Fortunately, most are quite benign and many are readily tolerated by patients. If a side-effect (for example, nausea, headache, cough, flushing, constipation) does occur and is troublesome, the doctor will usually switch to another drug. If it is extremely important to use a particular agent, then the side-effect may be treated in a specific way (for example, a laxative for constipation). For some drugs, periodic blood tests or electrocardiograms are needed to monitor for possible adverse effects that may not be noticed by the patient.

Some people experience discomforts with virtually every drug they receive. Often this is not due to the drug itself but to the person's dislike of being on medication. This presents a difficult problem for both the patient and the doctor. Some ways to deal with it are discussed in Chapter 15. Even with this problem, it is important to remember that blood pressure-lowering treatments reduce the complications of high blood pressure and that they can only work if taken regularly!

DIURETICS

S. George Carruthers, MD, and
C. R. Dean, MD

Diuretics (water pills) lower blood pressure by reducing the amount of water and salt in the body and relaxing the blood vessels. A low dose of a thiazide diuretic is a fairly common way of starting to treat mild or moderate hypertension. Together with beta-blockers (discussed in Chapters 6 and 8), they are recommended as initial (starting) treatment. They are convenient because they're taken once a day and are inexpensive. Diuretics are also useful for people who have heart failure.

How Diuretics Work

A diuretic increases the amount of salt and water that the kidneys remove from the body. The salt is sodium chloride, the same as regular table salt. The body acts very quickly to protect itself against the loss of too much water and salt, which could be harmful. After a few days there will be a new balance, with a little less water and salt in the body.

Your blood pressure will gradually decrease because there is a smaller volume of fluid in your circulation than before the diuretic was started. In addition, the amount of salt in the walls of the blood vessels decreases and causes them to dilate (or open up). This causes less resistance for the heart to pump against and helps the fall in blood pressure.

Diuretics tend to lower both systolic and diastolic blood pressure more effectively in older people. These drugs are favoured, therefore, in older people, including those with elevated diastolic and systolic blood pressure, and those with elevated systolic blood pressure with normal or low diastolic pressure (so-called "isolated" systolic hypertension).

Types of Diuretics

There are four main groups of diuretics: thiazides or thiazide-like diuretics, potassium-sparing diuretics, combination diuretics, and loop diuretics. Table 7-1 gives more details and examples of each group. Only commonly used diuretics have been mentioned. All drugs have both brand (trade) name(s) and a nonproprietary or generic name. Ask your doctor or pharmacist for the generic name if in doubt as to what kind of drug you're getting, because different companies make similar drugs under different brand names. Newer drugs usually have just one brand name and one generic name. Drugs that have been on the market for several years sometimes have two or more brand names. This is because they are manufactured by different companies. However, they still have only one generic name.

Thiazide Diuretics

The thiazide or thiazide-like diuretics are often known as thiazides for short. Their effect is usually mild, comes on gradually, and lasts a relatively long time. You may not notice any difference in the amount of urine you produce when you start taking them; just the same, most people prefer to take them in the morning to avoid having to get up in the middle of the night. This is the type of diuretic that is most often used in the treatment of mild to moderate hypertension. The thiazides are also commonly used in more severe hypertension. In this case they're given in combination with one or more of the other medicines described in this book such as beta-blockers (Chapter 8), ACE inhibitors (Chapter 9) or calcium antagonists (Chapter 10).

Table 7-1: Commonly Prescribed Diuretics

Class	Generic Name	Brand Name	Usual Daily Dose (mg)
Thiazide-like	Chlorthalidone	Hygroton	12.5–25
	Hydrochlorothiazide	Hydrodiuril Esidrix	12.5–50
	Indapamide	Lozide	2.5
Potassium-sparing	Amiloride	Midamor	★
	Spironolactone	Aldactone	25–100
	Triamterene	Dyrenium	★
Combination	Hydrochlorothiazide *plus*		
	Amiloride	Moduret	1–2 tablets
	Spironolactone	Aldactazide	1–2 tablets
	Triamterene	Dyazide	1–2 tablets
Loop	Furosemide	Lasix	20–80

★ These medications are rarely used alone.

Potassium-Sparing Diuretics

Potassium is an important mineral for the functioning of all body tissues. Thiazide and loop diuretics sometimes cause low potassium, which can lead to weakness or tiredness of the muscles and heart trouble. Potassium-sparing diuretics act on the kidneys in a different way from thiazides or loop diuretics. Sometimes these medications actually lead to an increase in potassium in the blood and tissues. They tend to be rather weak at lowering blood pressure, however, so they're not often used by themselves. Spironolactone is the exception, being used in some forms of high blood pressure that are associated with a lot of salt being held in the body or too great a loss of potassium.

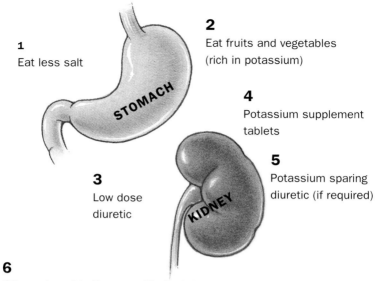

1
Eat less salt

2
Eat fruits and vegetables
(rich in potassium)

4
Potassium supplement
tablets

5
Potassium sparing
diuretic (if required)

3
Low dose
diuretic

6
If these steps 1 to 5 are not effective in keeping potassium level satisfactory, it
may be necessary to look for specific causes of excessive potassium loss.

Figure 7-1: Keeping potassium levels normal

In patients with poor kidneys and in patients who are taking other medications that keep potassium in the body, potassium-sparing drugs may cause the potassium level to increase
too much, a potentially dangerous situation. If potassium-sparing drugs are given at all in patients with poor renal function,
blood tests must be taken often to ensure that both potassium
and renal function remain acceptable (Fig. 7-1).

Combination Diuretics
These drugs are mixtures of a thiazide and one of the potassium-sparing medicines. They generally keep the blood level of
potassium normal. However, they tend to be more expensive
and usually cause little more lowering of blood pressure than
the thiazides alone.

Loop Diuretics
In contrast to thiazides, loop diuretics act very quickly. They
can cause a large loss of fluid over a short time. Shortly after

taking these pills, most people have to pass a lot of urine. Therefore, it's not a good idea to take such a tablet just before driving a car or going to the supermarket! Most people prefer taking this type of diuretic shortly after they get up in the morning so the effects have worn off before they go out.

In the hours after a dose of this type of diuretic has finished working, the body compensates for the salt and water losses by holding on to fluid, so there is little urine output for a while. Because of their large effect on urine output and the short duration of this effect, loop diuretics are usually prescribed for the treatment of high blood pressure only when there are other complications. They're very useful, however, in patients who have heart failure. They're also helpful when there is a decrease in kidney function. Sometimes they're used in combination with other medications in the treatment of severe hypertension.

Side-Effects of Diuretics

Most people do not experience any bad side-effects from using diuretics. However, diuretics can cause several chemical changes in the body that may lead to the following problems.

Increase in Blood Sugar

Diuretics increase blood sugar slightly in most people. Generally, this is not a problem, but in people with a tendency to develop diabetes, this increase in blood sugar may be enough to bring out the symptoms of diabetes. Any increase in thirst or passing larger amounts of urine after you have been taking a diuretic for a few weeks should be discussed with your doctor. In patients who already have diabetes, diuretics might make diabetes worse. The use of diuretics alone in such patients will generally be avoided, but they can be useful as add-on therapy.

Decrease in Blood Potassium (Hypokalemia)

Diuretics cause the loss not only of salt and water but also of other chemicals in the body (known as electrolytes) such as potassium and magnesium. If blood potassium decreases too much, your muscles will not function as well and you may feel tired. For patients with heart trouble, particularly those using the heart drug digoxin, the heart is very sensitive to a low level of blood potassium and may beat irregularly.

A small fall in potassium is not a serious matter unless you have heart disease and are on digoxin. Also, if the potassium is low, it can be treated easily, as we discuss below. If your potassium level falls a lot while you are on a small dose of thiazide, this may signal a problem with the blood supply to your kidneys or a disorder of the adrenal glands, and your doctor may decide to do some additional tests (see Chapters 1 and 2).

Increase in Blood Uric Acid

Uric acid is a chemical produced by the body and excreted in the urine. If too much stays in the body, it can cause gout. In this disease, crystals of uric acid make the lining of a joint inflamed and sore. Typically, gout shows up as a red, tender, painful big toe, but other joints can also be affected. Diuretics sometimes cause an increase in uric acid and can start an attack of gout in those who have a tendency to it. Fortunately, most people are not inclined that way. If the uric acid level in your body goes up a little, your doctor likely won't treat it. It usually doesn't lead to any harm. If you have an acute attack of gout, it may be necessary to stop your diuretic. Sometimes other medicines, such as allopurinol, are used to help cut down the amount of uric acid that your body makes.

Increase in Blood Cholesterol

Cholesterol is a fatty material that can be found in the blood. It's necessary for making some very important hormones and for making membranes that surround body cells. If the amount of cholesterol in the blood becomes too great for a long time, the arteries become thickened and hardened and there is an increased chance of heart attack. The level of cholesterol can be increased temporarily by diuretics. It is recommended that the blood cholesterol level be checked before medication is started. It might also be checked again after the treatment has been given for several months. If your doctor finds that your cholesterol level is too high, you may have to reduce your weight and make some changes in your diet or try another treatment for the high blood pressure.

Other Problems

Sometimes medications lower the blood pressure too much. This will first show up as dizziness upon standing. Sometimes men suffer from impotence, or a decrease in sexual function, after taking diuretics for a while. Occasionally, diuretics may cause too much fluid loss or dehydration. This can occur when the doses of the diuretics are too high. Dehydration may also occur in people who don't drink enough water and in people who sweat a lot in very hot weather. It may also occur in people with a bad attack of diarrhea. If you think you have any of those problems and may be dehydrated, you should drink some extra fluid and call your doctor. Rarely, diuretics can also cause a rash.

Preventing Side-Effects

What can we do about these side-effects? In recent years we have learned that low doses of thiazides work almost as well as larger doses for lowering blood pressure, and the chance of having most side-effects is much less at these lower doses. For example, doctors now prescribe as little as 12.5 mg daily of chlorthalidone or hydrochlorothiazide, instead of up to 100 mg a day as we once prescribed several years ago. We see hardly any side-effects at these low doses.

If side-effects do occur, the best approach is usually to stop the diuretic and try another medication to lower blood pressure. Sometimes, however, a patient needs a diuretic. For example, if someone has high blood pressure and heart failure, it may be necessary to relieve the heart by lowering the amount of fluid in the body. In such cases we may have to accept and treat a side-effect.

In heart patients, the decrease in blood potassium is a side-effect that we don't want. One way to prevent this is to eat foods rich in potassium and low in salt (most fresh fruits and vegetables, particularly bananas, oranges and potatoes). This also helps the diuretic do its job of lowering blood pressure. Another way to increase potassium in the body is to take potassium tablets or liquid. Potassium tablets or liquids can be expensive and large amounts may be necessary to get enough potassium into the body. A better and simpler way is to combine the regular diuretic with a potassium-sparing one (see "combination tablets" in Table 7-1). But even better, if you're concerned about low blood potassium, it's better to eat more fresh fruits and vegetables (see Chapter 4 for more information).

Although low doses of thiazide diuretics make the chance of these chemical changes much lower, the doctor will want to do blood tests from time to time to make sure that no important changes occur after you start these pills. This is one of the disadvantages of the diuretics and why some doctors and patients don't like using them. The extra laboratory tests do add to the cost, but diuretics are still very inexpensive unless many laboratory tests are done.

CHAPTER 8

DRUGS AND THE SYMPATHETIC NERVOUS SYSTEM

Jack Onrot, MD, and Tom Wilson, MD

In this chapter we'll discuss drugs that affect the sympathetic nervous system: beta-blockers, alpha-blockers and centrally acting agents, including clonidine and some older drugs, methyldopa, reserpine and guanethidine.

As explained in Chapter 1, the involuntary (or autonomic) nervous system plays an important role in the control of blood pressure. The autonomic nervous system is divided into two major parts, the parasympathetic and the sympathetic nervous systems. The sympathetic system produces the well-known

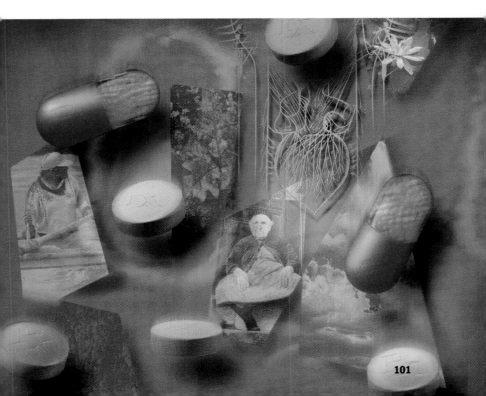

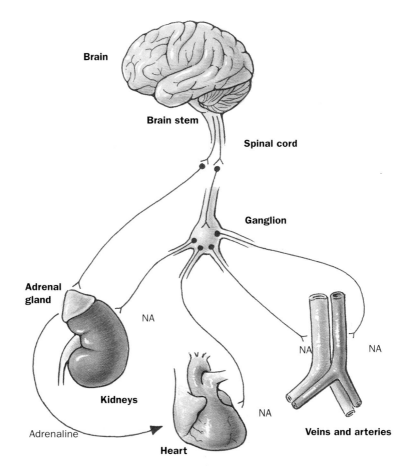

Figure 8-1: The sympathetic nervous system

fight-or-flight response that occurs when a person is in a threatening situation. By blocking the activity of this system, certain drugs can lower blood pressure. The sympathetic nervous system is controlled by the brain stem, the lowest part of the brain, located just above the spinal cord at the top of the neck. Sympathetic nerve impulses travel from the brain stem down the spinal cord, and they transfer their information to nerve fibres that travel to the heart, blood vessels and other important tissues, as shown in Figure 8-1.

Nerve impulses are tiny electrical signals. Sympathetic

nerve impulses cause the nerve ending to release noradrena-line. The noradrenaline crosses a small gap to the adjacent tissues in the heart, kidney or blood vessels and binds to special receptors located there. There are two types of receptors for noradrenaline, called alpha and beta. Beta-1 receptors in the heart, when activated by noradrenaline, cause the heart to beat faster and more strongly, thus raising blood pressure. Stimulation of alpha receptors in the blood vessels by noradrenaline causes the vessels to narrow, again raising blood pressure. On the other hand, stimulation of beta-2 receptors in blood vessels causes them to open up, lowering the blood pressure. Adrenaline, from the adrenal gland, circulates in the blood and also activates these receptors (this is outlined in Fig. 8-2). Finally, impulses from the sympathetic nerves can stimulate the production of renin by the kidney, leading to increased blood pressure (see Chapter 9).

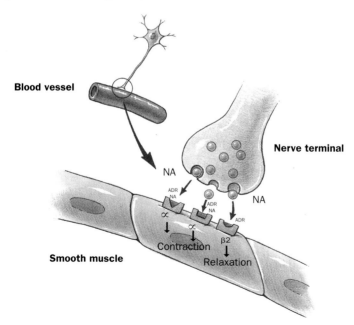

Figure 8-2: Sympathetic nerve terminal at a blood vessel

Blocking beta-1 receptors opposes the sympathetic nervous system activity in the heart and kidney, resulting in lower blood pressure. This is the basis of action of a group of drugs called beta-blockers.

Beta-Blockers

The various beta-blockers, their brand names, usual dosages and types of action are listed in Table 8-1. Beta-blockers block the action of noradrenaline and adrenaline at beta-receptors, reducing the force and speed of contraction of the heart and decreasing renin secretion by the kidney, leading to reductions in blood pressure.

Beta-blockers tend to be more effective in younger patients than in those over 65 years of age. They're also less effective in

Table 8-1 Characteristics of Beta-Blockers

Generic Name	Brand Name	Usual Daily Dosage (mg)	Beta-1 Selective	Water-Soluble	ISA*
Acebutolol	Monitan	200-800	+	+	+
	Sectral	200-800	+	+	+
Atenolol	Tenormin	25-100	+	+	−
Labetalol	Trandate	200-800	−	−	−
Metoprolol	Betaloc	25-200	−	−	−
	Lopresor	25-200	+	−	−
Nadolol	Corgard	20-80	−	+	−
Oxprenolol	Trasicor	60-320	−	−	+
Pindolol	Visken	5-30	−	−	+
Propranolol	Inderal	40-320	−	−	−
Timolol	Blocadren	5-40	−	−	−

* intrinsic sympathomimetic activity (mild stimulant effect).

+ drug has this property.

− drug does not have this property.

black patients. Beta-blockers are useful for people in whom high sympathetic nervous system activity is suspected, such as very anxious patients or patients who have relatively high heart rates. Beta-blockers are used in many other medical conditions, and when these conditions coexist with hypertension, it is clearly an advantage to use beta-blockers to treat all of the coexisting problems. Table 8-2 gives a brief list of conditions that will benefit or suffer from the use of beta-blockers. Note that these are guidelines only. Your doctor will take other factors into account in making the decision about whether a beta-blocker should be prescribed.

There are also conditions for which beta-blockers may be harmful including asthma, severe heart failure, and severe blockage of the arteries to the limbs ("claudication"). The "Avoid if" column of Table 8-2 is a list of potential reasons to avoid using beta-blockers. Please note that beta-blockers may still do more good than harm even if a person has some of the "Avoid if" conditions. For example, if a person has mild

Table 8-2: Some Factors Influencing Choice of Beta-Blockers

Choose if	Avoid if
Previous heart attack	Asthma/emphysema
Angina	Raynaud's phenomenon
Rapid heart rhythms	Peripheral artery blockage (claudication)
Migraines	Diabetes
Tremor	Slow heart rhythms
Anxiety	Heart failure
Overactive thyroid	Depression
Glaucoma	Impotence
Aneurysm of aorta	Elevated cholesterol/triglycerides
	Chronic fatigue
	Sleep disturbances
	Exercise intolerance

cramps in their legs from blockage of the blood supply, beta-blockers may not make this worse, and so could be used to treat hypertension in this case. Doctors may prescribe beta-blockers for patients with such conditions, but will watch carefully for adverse effects. Should you suspect that you have one of these problems, or if you feel your beta-blocker is causing other problems, be sure to discuss it with your doctor.

Beta-receptors in the heart differ somewhat from those located elsewhere. *Selective* beta-blockers such as atenolol (Tenormin), metoprolol (Betaloc, Lopresor) and acebutolol (Monitan, Sectral) are so-named because they block beta-1 receptors in the heart more than beta-2 receptors elsewhere. It's sometimes advantageous to avoid blocking noncardiac beta-2 receptors because they can open up blood vessels and air tubes (*bronchi*) to the lung. Blocking this beta-2 "opening up" action with beta-blockers worsens asthma or reduces circulation to the fingers and legs. In the case of asthma, none of the beta-blockers is safe and therefore should be avoided.

Beta-blockers may cause side-effects even if the user has no "Avoid if" conditions. They can cause fatigue and decreased ability to exercise and can interfere with sexual function, causing decreased libido (sex drive) and impotence. They may also disturb sleep. Fortunately, these side-effects are not common and disappear when the drug is stopped.

Some beta-blockers mildly stimulate beta receptors; this effect goes by the tongue-twisting name *intrinsic sympathomimetic activity*. Examples are acebutolol (Monitan, Sectral), pindolol (Visken), and oxprenolol (Trasicor). These drugs are useful in treating patients who have low heart rates. They may also have advantages over other beta-blockers in the treatment of hypertensive patients with high cholesterol since this group of beta-blockers does not increase cholesterol.

Some beta-blockers dissolve better in water than in fat (that is, they are water-soluble) whereas other beta-blockers dissolve better in fat than water (that is, they are lipid-soluble). Because the barrier separating the brain's circulation from the body's circulation is made of lipids, lipid-soluble beta-blockers tend to enter the brain more easily. Certain beta-blocker side-effects are due to the entry of the drug into the brain. They include nightmares, depression, fatigue and impotence. These problems occur less often with the water-soluble beta-blockers, which include nadolol (Corgard), atenolol (Tenormin), and acebutolol (Monitan, Sectral).

A unique drug, labetalol (Trandate), has both beta- and mild alpha-blocking activity, which provides additional blood pressure lowering. For more information, see the next section on alpha-blockers.

Alpha-Blockers

Alpha-blockers, including doxazosin (Cardura), prazosin (Minipress) and terazosin (Hytrin), hinder the action of noradrenaline and adrenaline at alpha-receptors on blood vessels. Because noradrenaline and adrenaline narrow blood vessels through their action on alpha-receptors, blocking their action will relax blood vessels and lower blood pressure.

Alpha-blockers can be used alone for hypertension, but they are usually used in combination with other drugs. They often lose some degree of effectiveness with prolonged use. Combining these agents with other drugs, such as diuretics (Chapter 7), can prevent or reduce this gradual loss of effectiveness.

Alpha-blockers have one advantage over all other antihypertensive agents in that they actually lower cholesterol in the blood. Although this effect is moderate, it may be important in patients with already elevated cholesterol levels. Most of the other drugs have no effect on cholesterol, but certain classes may raise cholesterol, for example, diuretics in high doses and nonselective beta-blockers.

A small percentage of patients will have a profound fall in

blood pressure and may even faint following the first dose of an alpha-blocker or after an increase in dose. This is known as the *first-dose effect*. Although this effect is rare, it can be minimized by giving a small initial dose (0.5 mg) and starting it at bedtime, when the person is unlikely to be getting up within the next 2 or 3 hours. It should be emphasized that this first-dose effect is encountered only when taking the first pill or when the dosage is increased. Other side-effects sometimes occur, including fatigue, light-headedness, headaches and upset stomach.

Drugs That Work in the Brain (Centrally Acting Drugs)

Table 8-3 lists drugs other than beta-blockers that act on the sympathetic nervous system.

Clonidine (Catapres) and methyldopa (Aldomet) act in the brain to reduce the flow of messages from the brain through sympathetic nerves. This lowers the blood pressure. These drugs have the advantage that they have no adverse effects on lipids or electrolytes (such as potassium) in the blood. Unfortunately, because they act in the brain, they can cause fatigue, sedation, or even confusion. These drugs may also cause impotence in men, reduction of libido in men and women, dry mouth and

Generic Name	Brand Name	Usual Daily Dosage (mg)	Type
Doxazosin	Cardura	1-8	Alpha-blocker
Prazosin	Minipress	1.0–20	Alpha-blocker
Terazosin	Hytrin	1.0–20	Alpha-blocker
Clonidine	Catapres	0.1–1.2	Central agent
Methyldopa	Aldomet	250–2,000	Central agent
Reserpine	Serpasil	0.05–0.5	Noradrenaline depletor

Table 8-3: Other Agents That Affect Sympathetic Activity

stuffy nose. Because the sympathetic nervous system is essential for maintaining blood pressure when we stand up, these agents may cause upright blood pressures to become too low. This produces light-headedness or even fainting. Methyldopa has a slow and long-acting effect. In contrast, clonidine acts quickly and also disappears quickly. Stopping clonidine suddenly can cause rapid heart beat, a feeling of anxiety, and very high blood pressure readings. It is important not to run out of your prescription. If the drug must be stopped, it should be done over a period of several days.

Drugs That Act on Sympathetic Nerve Endings

Two drugs, reserpine (Serpasil) and guanethidine (Ismelin), act on sympathetic nerves. Their side-effects are similar to those of the centrally acting agents but are much more frequent. Guanethidine, because of its side-effects, is seldom used.

Reserpine depletes nerves of noradrenaline. It is one of the oldest known antihypertensive drugs but fell out of favour because of its tendency to cause depression. However, depression can be avoided by using low doses. Some doctors favour the use of reserpine in selected patients, because it has no adverse effects on lipids or electrolytes. It can also be given once a day, is often quite effective in small doses, and is inexpensive.

Conclusions

All the drugs described in this chapter share the common characteristic of reducing, in one way or another, sympathetic nervous system activity. The drugs that work outside the brain (beta-and alpha-blockers) have fewer side-effects than centrally acting drugs, and thus are often preferred by patients and their doctors. Nevertheless, centrally acting drugs are effective in lowering blood pressure and are often well tolerated by patients, particularly in low doses.

ACE INHIBITORS

Louise F. Roy, MD, and

Frans H. H. Leenen, MD, PhD

Angiotensin converting enzyme inhibitors or ACE inhibitors (it's easy to see why the name has been shortened!) are an important group of blood pressure-lowering drugs. They work by inhibiting the actions of the renin-angiotensin system. As described in Chapters 1 and 2, the renin-angiotensin system helps in the regulation of normal blood pressure. In hypertension, the system may work at a level that is too high, raising the blood pressure above normal. The renin-angiotensin system is shown in Figure 9-1.

The first step in this system is renin, an enzyme produced by the kidneys. Renin transforms a protein (angiotensinogen) into a smaller molecule, angiotensin I. Angiotensin I is transformed into Angiotensin II by another enzyme, angiotensin-converting enzyme (ACE). Angiotensin II is a potent hormone that narrows blood vessels. This increases the resistance of the vessels to blood flow and thus increases the blood pressure.

The main effect of ACE inhibitors is to decrease the effect of the angiotensin-converting enzyme. The result is easy to predict: decreased production of angiotensin II. Figure 9-2 shows how, in the presence of ACE inhibitors, the quantity of angiotensin II in the blood will decrease. This results in a decrease in the resistance of blood vessels and lowers the blood pressure.

ACE inhibitors don't change heart rate or heart function. However, because they decrease vessel resistance and blood pressure, they decrease the amount of work that the heart has to perform. This improves heart activity in patients with heart failure.

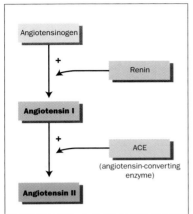

FIGURE 9-1: Renin-angiotensin system

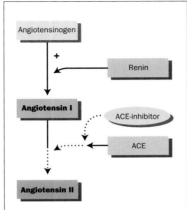

Figure 9-2: Renin-angiotensin system with ACE inhibitor

Table 9-1: ACE Inhibitors

Generic Name	Brand Name	Starting Dose (mg)	Average Daily Dose (mg)	Frequency of Administration (times per day)
Benazepril	Lotensin	10	10–40	1
Captopril	Capoten	6.25–25	25–100	2–4
Cilazapril	Inhibace	2–5	5–10	1
Enalapril	Vasotec	2.5–5	5–20	1–2
Fosinopril	Monopril	10	10–40	1
Lisinopril	Prinivil	5-10	10–40	1
	Zestril	5-10	10–40	1
Perindopril	Coversyl	2	4-8	1
Quinapril	Accupril	10	10-40	1
Ramipril	Altace	2.5	2.5–20	1

There are many ACE inhibitors available in Canada; Table 9-1 shows some of their characteristics.

When ACE Inhibitors Are Used

ACE inhibitors may be used alone or in combination with other antihypertensive drugs. ACE inhibitors are not equally effective in all patients. For example, black people respond less well to them than white people. On the other hand, in patients taking diuretics (water pills), or on salt-restricted diets, ACE inhibitors are efficient blood pressure-lowering drugs. This is because the renin-angiotensin system is more active in these situations.

Patients suffering from heart failure, whether or not they have high blood pressure, often have increased activity of the renin-angiotensin system. ACE inhibitors may improve their symptoms of heart failure and improve their quality of life. Overall, ACE inhibitors are very effective for these patients. Large decreases in blood pressure may occur, however, so it's usual to start these patients on low doses.

Diabetics sometimes develop kidney disease. ACE inhibitors seem to be more effective than other blood pressure-lowering drugs in slowing the progression of kidney damage.

Hypertension is sometimes caused by a narrowing of an artery that provides blood to one of the kidneys, causing increased production of renin. In this case, ACE inhibitors also effectively lower blood pressure, particularly when used with a diuretic (refer to Chapter 7).

When ACE Inhibitors Are Avoided

The renin-angiotensin system plays an important role in the function of the kidneys. Because they inhibit the renin-angiotensin system, ACE inhibitors can impair the function of the kidneys. For this reason when the arteries to *both* kidneys are narrowed, ACE inhibitors should not be used.

Some patients may retain potassium because of a decrease in its excretion by the kidneys. This occurs most often when kidney function is poor. ACE inhibitors can aggravate this situation and should not be used in this circumstance.

Some drugs should not be used together with ACE inhibitors or must be used very carefully. These include potassium supplements, anti-inflammatory drugs (used in arthritis), and a special group of diuretics that cause potassium retention.

Side-Effects of ACE Inhibitors

As mentioned, ACE inhibitors may decrease kidney function and cause potassium accumulation if kidney function is poor. As well, they can produce large decreases in blood pressure in some patients. Fortunately, these effects are reversible and once the drug is discontinued, organ and body functions will revert to previous levels.

A dry cough may occur in 5% to 10% of patients; this is more common if lung disease is already present. Skin rashes occur in 2% to 4% of patients within the first 2 or 3 months. In 1% to 2% of patients, there is a decrease in taste or a metallic-sour taste. Very rarely, the number of white blood cells may decrease.

Angioedema is a rare but important side-effect that can happen in the first month. This is an allergic reaction and includes swelling of the mouth, lips and throat. *This is dangerous: at the first sign call a doctor immediately!*

All these side-effects are reversible and will disappear if the drug is stopped soon enough. ACE inhibitors should not be used during pregnancy, however, as malformed babies have been reported when pregnant women have taken this drug.

CHAPTER 10

CALCIUM ANTAGONISTS

Louise F. Roy, MD, and
Frans H. H. Leenen, MD, PhD

Calcium antagonists, also known as calcium channel-blockers, are a class of drugs that work by interfering with the entry of calcium into cells (Fig. 10-1). Calcium plays many roles inside the cells of the body. In blood vessel walls, calcium influences muscle cell contraction. To do so, it has to enter these cells through tiny channels in the cell walls. Calcium antagonists interfere with this entry of calcium into the cells. Hence, calcium antagonists relax the muscle in vessel walls, decreasing resistance to blood flow and blood pressure. They act as vasodilators (or "vessel dilators") as described in Chapter 11(see Fig. 11-1).

However, calcium antagonists differ from other vasodilators in two important ways. First, they partially block signals from the nerves to the heart. This lessens the increase in heart rate that usually happens with vasodilators other than calcium antagonists. Second, calcium antagonists have a small diuretic effect (see Chapter 7 for more on diuretics). The kidneys are less likely to retain fluid, a problem caused by other vasodilators. Therefore, calcium antagonists have some advantages over other vasodilators.

In fact, calcium antagonists have many ideal features for lowering blood pressure. Compared with some other blood pressure-lowering drugs such as diuretics, they don't have undesirable effects on blood lipids (cholesterol and triglycerides), blood potassium, sodium (salt), uric acid or glucose (blood sugar). More recent studies have shown that calcium antagonists may also have a beneficial, preventive effect on the development of atherosclerosis (hardening of the arteries caused by deposits of lipids and calcium in the walls of arter-

Table 10-1: Calcium Antagonists

Generic Name	Brand Name	Starting Dose (mg)	Average Daily Dose (mg)	Frequency of Administration (times per day)
Amlodipine	Norvasc	2.5–5	5–10	1
Diltiazem	Cardizem	30	90–360	3–4
	Cardizem SR	60	120–360	2
	Cardizem CD	120	120–360	1
Felodipine	Plendil	2.5–5	5–10	1
	Renedil	2.5–5	5–10	1
Nicardipine	Cardene	20	60–120	3
Nifedipine	Adalat PA	10–20	20–120	2–3
	Adalat XL	30	30–120	1
Verapamil	Isoptin	80	240–480	3
	Isoptin SR	120	240–480	1–2

ies). Table 10-1 shows the calcium antagonists currently available in Canada, both in regular and long-acting form.

Calcium antagonists can be separated into two classes. The drugs ending in "...dipine" (such as nifedipine) are more vasodilating and less heart-slowing, whereas others (verapamil and diltiazem) are more heart-slowing and have less vasodilating effect.

When Calcium Antagonists Are Used

In addition to their benefits for lowering blood pressure, calcium antagonists are useful for the treatment of angina. This is because they decrease the activity of the heart and therefore its work. Thus, for patients with both angina and high blood pressure, they may be a good choice. Calcium antagonists have been shown to be more effective in patients with low renin

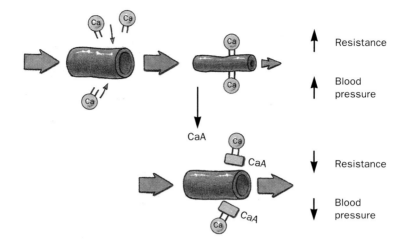

Figure 10-1: Mechanism of action of calcium antagonists (CaA)

(for a brief description of the renin-angiotensin system, see Chapters 1 or 9). This includes elderly and black people.

As the "...dipine" calcium antagonists may accelerate the heart rate, their use with a beta-blocker is a good choice, provided the heart function is relatively normal (beta-blockers are described in Chapter 8).

Calcium antagonists are also useful in lowering blood pressure when certain drugs (such as diuretics or beta-blockers) must be avoided because the patient has other medical conditions (for example, asthma, high cholesterol/triglyceride levels, gout, Raynaud's disease, or diabetes).

When Calcium Antagonists Are Avoided

Currently available calcium antagonists may decrease the strength and frequency of heart contractions. If the heart is failing, these calcium antagonists can make this worse.

Verapamil and diltiazem should be used very carefully with beta-blockers. If they're combined with a beta-blocker, the electrical conduction in the heart may be slowed too much. Patients with prior problems with the electrical (impulse) conducting system of the heart should not be prescribed the currently available calcium antagonists, as their condition may worsen.

Side-Effects of Calcium Antagonists

The "...dipine" calcium antagonists act a little like a vasodilator and can cause headaches, palpitations and flushing. These symptoms will usually decrease within a few weeks. The short-acting forms of these drugs more often cause these side-effects, as the drug is rapidly absorbed and its quantity in the blood increases suddenly. The more long-acting forms are absorbed slowly. The quantity of drug in the blood doesn't peak as much and remains more constant. In either case, use with a beta-blocker may prevent some of these side-effects.

Calcium antagonists, particularly the "...dipines", may cause ankle swelling. This is not due to water retention, as some of these drugs have a small diuretic effect on their own; rather it's because of an effect on the small blood vessels. Therefore, adding a diuretic will not help.

Calcium antagonists may cause digestive disorders such as nausea, heartburn and, infrequently, a decrease in appetite or diarrhea. Verapamil is particularly associated with constipation.

Fortunately, all these side-effects are reversible by discontinuing use of the drug.

CHAPTER 11

VASODILATORS

Louise F. Roy, MD, and
Frans H. H. Leenen, MD, PhD

Vasodilators relax the muscle of the blood vessel walls. The vessels dilate and the resistance to the flow of blood within them decreases (Fig. 11-1). If this dilation were the only effect, these drugs would be well suited for the treatment of high blood pressure. Unfortunately, they have several other effects that counteract their blood pressure-lowering effect. They cause the kidneys to retain sodium (salt) and water, so the total water and sodium in the body increases. They also cause the heart to beat faster and more strongly. These last two consequences tend to partly overcome the beneficial effect of relaxing the blood vessels.

In hypertension, the heart has to pump harder to overcome the higher resistance. Gradually it becomes larger. This increase in heart size (or heart hypertrophy) increases the risk of complications such as heart failure and sudden death. Fortunately, the heart size may return to normal if high blood pressure is treated well. However, vasodilators used alone will make the heart work even harder so that the heart size may not return to normal and may even get worse.

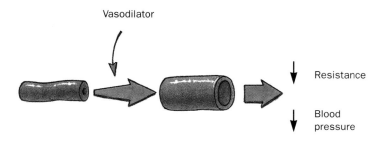

Figure 11-1: Mechanism of action of vasodilators

Table 11-1: Common Vasodilators Used in Canada			
Generic Name	Brand Name	Average Daily Dose (mg)	Frequency of Administration (times per day)
Hydralazine	Apresoline	50–200	2–3
Minoxidil	Loniten	2.5–20	1–2

Two vasodilators that can be taken by mouth, hydralazine and minoxidil, are available in Canada for the treatment of high blood pressure (Table 11-1). Other vasodilators are used only intravenously in the hospital.

When Vasodilators Are Used

Vasodilators usually aren't used alone. They're most often given with a beta-blocker and a diuretic to overcome the side-effects of vasodilators on the kidneys and the heart, described above.

Hydralazine is one of the few drugs that can be used safely by pregnant hypertensive patients.

Minoxidil is a potent drug to lower pressure. It's particularly helpful when the blood pressure is very high and has been difficult to control with other drugs. Once the blood pressure settles down, other drugs are usually substituted, but sometimes it's necessary to continue with minoxidil.

When Vasodilators Are Avoided

Vasodilators increase the work of the heart, making it beat faster and more powerfully. If you have angina, vasodilators may worsen it.

In recent years, we've seen the development of new classes of drugs that are easier to use and have fewer side-effects.

These drugs, such as calcium antagonists and ACE inhibitors, are replacing vasodilators.

Side-Effects of Vasodilators

Headache, flushing and palpitations are frequent side-effects of vasodilators. These are sometimes temporary problems and disappear gradually by themselves or when the vasodilators are combined with beta-blockers. Vasodilators, when used alone, may worsen angina. Ankle swelling is another side-effect and is due to the retention of salt and water by the kidneys; a diuretic may counteract this.

In high doses (300 mg or more per day), hydralazine may cause the patient to produce antibodies against his own body, resulting in painful, swollen joints. This is reversible, provided the drug was not used for too long.

Minoxidil may increase hair growth on the body. In fact, it's now made into an ointment to rub on the scalp to help with some forms of baldness. Bald people should use this ointment only if they have normal heart function, because some of the minoxidil is absorbed from the scalp and may increase the activity of the heart. In rare cases, water may accumulate in the envelope (pericardium) around the heart. These side-effects are reversible if minoxidil is stopped.

CHAPTER 12

HYPERTENSION IN THE ELDERLY

Pierre Larochelle, MD, PhD,
and A. Mark Clarfield, MD

High blood pressure is considered to be a major risk factor for the development of heart and vascular diseases in older individuals. There is no set definition of being "older", for example 65 years. Studies that have looked at hypertension or other diseases have used age groups such as 60 to 74 years, 75 to 84 years and over 85 years to help us to understand the risks of high blood pressure and benefits and risks of treatment in relation to age.

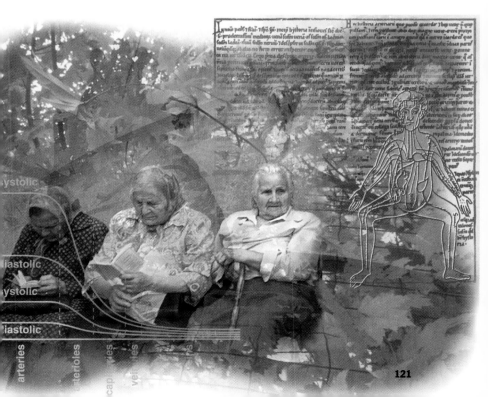

For the elderly, average blood pressures of more than 140 mm Hg systolic and 90 mm Hg diastolic (140/90 mm Hg) are a matter of concern. At this level of blood pressure, there is a significant increase in the risk of future cardiovascular disease. This does not necessarily mean that drug treatment has to be started at this level. However, the higher the pressure, the higher the risk, and the more likely your doctor will start treatment.

The incidence of hypertension increases with age. Fifty six per cent of men and 52% of women over the age of 65 years have a blood pressure higher than it should be. The systolic pressure (the higher number) in particular increases with age. Although it was once thought that the diastolic pressure (the low number) was more important, in older people the systolic pressure indicates the level of risk slightly better. Thus, the systolic pressure is now given more weight in deciding when to treat.

In some cases, the systolic pressure can increase without any change in the diastolic pressure (for example, 170/80 mm Hg). This type of high blood pressure is called isolated systolic hypertension.

The blood pressure of persons over the age of 65 years should be checked at least once a year. If it is higher than 140 mm Hg, then more frequent readings are taken by a nurse or a physician to determine a proper course of action. Only if the blood pressure remains high may treatment be needed.

Hypertension and Cardiovascular Risk Factors

There are a number of factors that can lead to cardiac disease (heart failure, heart attack), stroke or an aneurysm (a weakening and swelling of the aorta, which is the major blood vessel of the body). In younger people the major risk factors are cigarette smoking, high blood cholesterol and high blood pressure. In older people high blood pressure becomes the most treatable risk factor for heart or vascular disease. (*Smokers*: this doesn't mean you can continue to smoke! Stopping smoking is beneficial at any age.) The risk associated with an increased blood pressure is in fact greater in the elderly patient than the younger patient. The rise in blood pressure and increased prevalence of hypertension in the elderly are not harmless and should not be viewed as a normal consequence of aging.

Effects of High Blood Pressure on the Body

High blood pressure itself causes no complaints or symptoms in its early stages. However, if the high blood pressure is severe or remains untreated for a long time, damage to the heart, kidneys or brain may develop. For example, damage to the heart may cause shortness of breath, swelling of the feet, getting up more frequently during the night to pass urine, and sometimes pain in the chest (angina). Less often, these complaints can also occur in persons who have a normal blood pressure. When they are present, it is important to visit your physician.

Causes of High Blood Pressure

Hypertension can be divided according to its causes. Most persons (90–95%) with high blood pressure have "essential" hypertension. This term means that we do not really know what has caused the high blood pressure. It is likely that the hypertension is due to a combination of factors, such as dietary, environmental and genetic abnormalities. The other 5% to 10% of hypertensives have a "secondary" form of hypertension that is caused by dysfunction of the kidneys, the adrenal glands or of the blood vessels themselves (see Chapters 1 and 2 for more details).

In those over age 65, additional factors come into play. The most important is a change in the structure of the major blood vessels. These become less elastic and more rigid. This increased rigidity leads to an increase in the systolic blood pressure and plays the major role in the high prevalence of hypertension in this age group.

An isolated increase in the systolic pressure (> 160/80) occurs in 8% of those aged 60 to 69 years, 11% of those aged 70 to 79 years and 22% of those over the age of 80 years. There is also a decline in the function of the kidneys.

Investigation and Diagnosis

The investigation of hypertension is discussed fully in Chapter 2. The main difference in the elderly is the greater prevalence of high blood pressure. The diagnosis of high blood pressure is made when the reading is at least 140/90 mm Hg on at least three different occasions, a minimum of 1 week apart. This level of blood pressure indicates a need for special attention but may not mean that medical treatment is needed. When the diagnosis is made, a detailed physical examination should be made by your doctor to determine the condition of your heart and blood vessels. Laboratory tests will include urine and blood samples to evaluate the functions of your kidneys, and the blood sugar level as well as an electrocardiogram and possibly a chest x-ray.

Benefits of Treatment

It has been proven that 65- to 80-year-olds with hypertension who have their blood pressure lowered by medications suffer fewer strokes and are less likely to have heart failure than those who do not receive medication. In fact, studies indicate that this benefit is greater than in younger hypertensives.

Nevertheless, drug treatment is not without adverse effects. Thus, the risks and benefits of treatment have to be weighed for each person. Patients with milder hypertension (systolic readings between 140 and 160 mm Hg) may only require observation without treatment unless the physical examination or blood tests reveal damage to the brain, heart, kidneys or blood vessels. If you are over 80 years of age, the balance of benefits and risks of treatment have not been so clearly established. Depending on your other medical conditions, the physician may delay treatment to observe your condition before prescribing medications. He or she may even decide against drug treatment altogether.

Treatment is known to be generally beneficial for isolated systolic hypertension, as shown by large, careful studies. Treatment is now recommended for persons with a systolic pressure over 160 mm Hg. Each person, however, has unique circumstances and preferences and your physician will help you to evaluate the benefits and the risk of treatment in your case. Your medical history and symptoms, physical examination and laboratory tests will be considered along with the results of your blood pressure readings when you and your doctor decide on the treatment you should receive. For some people who experience adverse effects of medication, the potential benefits may not outweigh the possible harm particularly if the blood pressure is not too elevated.

Treatments

Treatments can be divided up into non-drug and drug therapies. Unfortunately, there are few studies of non-drug treatments in the elderly, and we are forced to use indirect evidence and guess whether the studies of non-drug therapy in younger people apply.

Non-Drug Therapies

Studies in the general population indicate that obesity is associated with an increased blood pressure, and in younger patients weight reduction can reduce blood pressure. Because of the difficulty of losing weight for older individuals, however, they are advised instead to follow a balanced diet and to maintain their present weight.

Consuming over 2 ounces (60 mL) of alcoholic beverages per day is associated with increased blood pressure, and alcohol should be restricted if your pressure is high.

Exercise is also generally healthy. As much as possible, walking or other forms of aerobic exercise should be used to "stay in shape" and may be helpful to control blood pressure (Chapter 5). If you wish to increase your level of exercise, your doctor can advise you and supervise your plans.

Salt should be reduced in the diet as much as is practical, because high salt intake is associated with increased blood pressure and a decrease in effectiveness of medications in lowering blood pressure.

Obviously smoking should be stopped as it causes further damage to your heart and blood vessels. The importance of reducing cholesterol levels is not known in older individuals, although very high levels probably should be reduced when possible. There is more complete information about non-drug treatments for hypertension in Chapters 4 and 5.

Medication

Patients over the age of 65 years who need drug treatment for their high blood pressure are usually prescribed the same medications as younger patients. As discussed in Chapter 6, a diuretic (or water pill) is usually preferred to start treatment for high blood pressure in the elderly. However, the choice of treatment also depends on several other factors (see Chapter 6).

In order to limit side-effects, the lowest possible dose will be prescribed. Indeed, one of the main goals in treating hypertensive patients over 65 years is ensuring that the blood pressure is brought as close as possible to normal levels without causing intolerable or dangerous adverse effects. If you have an abnormal reaction to a medication, you should notify your physician promptly so that a reduction or change in the medication can be considered. You should not stop taking the medication without advising your physician because a sudden and dangerous rise in blood pressure could result.

Summary

It should be remembered that a higher than normal blood pressure in an older person contributes to the risk of cardio-vascular disease. This risk increases as the level of the blood pressure rises and as the length of time that a person has had hypertension increases. Treatment can be useful to reduce the incidence of these complications. Nevertheless, the decision to treat and the choice of treatment must be individualized, taking into account your age, the level of blood pressure, other medical problems, any medications that you are already taking, and how well you tolerate BP medications.

CHAPTER 13

HYPERTENSION IN DIABETICS

Pavel Hamet, MD, PhD, and Jean-Hughes Brossard, MD

Diabetes is a disease in which the quantity of sugar (glucose) in the blood is elevated. Blood sugar is maintained at a stable level by the action of several hormones. One of these, insulin, is secreted by the pancreas. If the pancreas doesn't produce enough insulin, the blood sugar goes up (Type 1 diabetes). If the body produces insulin but the insulin doesn't work properly, the blood sugar also rises (Type 2 diabetes).

Type 1 diabetes (also called *insulin-dependent diabetes*) usually starts at a young age, in people below 30 years old. Type 2 diabetes (also called *non–insulin-dependent diabetes*) usually starts later in life, after 30 years of age. People with this problem still produce insulin, sometimes excessively. However, for various reasons including obesity, their insulin is less able to decrease blood sugar. Moreover, the quantity of insulin produced can also diminish with age.

Treating Diabetes

Diabetes treatment begins with diet. For Type 2 diabetics, medication that lowers blood sugar (called *oral hypoglycemic agents* — hypoglycemia means low blood sugar) may also be required. Insulin injections (one or more per day) are needed for all Type 1 diabetics and for some people with Type 2 diabetes.

There are two main goals of treatment. The first is to prevent life-threatening high blood sugar. High levels of sugar in the blood can lead to coma (unconsciousness); before the discovery of insulin, this was often fatal for Type 1 diabetics.

The second goal is to keep blood sugar levels as normal as possible. Strict control of blood sugar prevents late complications, which can be a consequence of either Types 1 or 2 diabetes.

Late Complications of Diabetes

With time, diabetes affects blood vessels at two levels. When large arteries are affected, the complications are called *macrovascular*. When the small vessels (arterioles and capillaries) are affected, the complications are *microvascular*.

Macrovascular Complications

Diseased large arteries progressively obstruct blood flow to the heart (coronary arteries), brain and legs. Symptoms vary, depending on the site of obstruction. They include angina and heart attack when the coronary arteries are affected, strokes when the brain arteries are obstructed, and cramps in the legs (claudication) on exercise when the leg arteries are narrowed. Other arteries can also become clogged including arteries to the kidneys, causing kidney (renal) failure, and to the penis, causing impotence.

Microvascular Complications

Obstruction of small vessels (also known as *microangiopathy*) mainly affects the eyes and kidneys. The retina, at the back of the eye, is most affected by diabetes. Damage to the retina is called retinopathy. It's a serious complication of diabetes and causes 25% of all new cases of blindness. Obstruction of small vessels in the kidney eventually causes kidney (renal) failure.

Hypertension in Diabetes

Close to 50% of diabetics have high blood pressure too (Fig. 13-1), and about 15% of hypertensive patients have problems

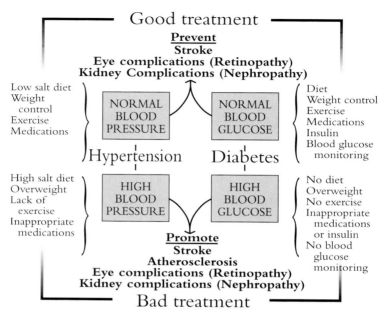

Figure 13-1: Diabetes and hypertension

with elevated blood sugar. The combination of hypertension and diabetes increases the chances of developing the complications described above. Furthermore, once complications are present, hypertension in diabetics increases the severity.

Two types of hypertension can be distinguished in diabetes: essential hypertension, and hypertension associated with renal disease (*nephropathy*). Essential hypertension in diabetics is probably of the same origin as in nondiabetics. Nevertheless, it has been demonstrated that diabetics have a greater tendency to retain salt and to more constriction of blood vessels. Both factors will contribute to higher blood pressures.

In nephropathy, the kidney doesn't function normally, and proteins are leaked from the blood into the urine. Hypertension in this situation is generally attributed to the renal disease. Thus, renal disease in diabetics leads to hypertension, and hypertension on its own can worsen the renal problem. This is a vicious circle with serious consequences. It can also be a warning sign of retinopathy. With special laboratory tests, we can recognize at an early stage who is at risk of developing these diabetic complications.

Benefits of Controlling Hypertension

There are many advantages in strictly controlling hypertension in diabetics. Several studies have demonstrated that hypertension therapy decreases protein losses in urine and slows the rate of kidney function deterioration. In this way, the vicious circle can be broken. Good control of hypertension in diabetics also decreases the risk of stroke and the progression of retinopathy.

When Hypertension Should Be Treated

All diabetics with diastolic blood pressure exceeding 100 mm Hg benefit from antihypertensive medication. If any vascular complications, including retinopathy and nephropathy, are detected, it's preferable to treat diastolic blood pressures of 90 mm Hg or higher to slow their progression. Indeed, many doctors believe that all diabetics with diastolic pressure at or above 90 mm Hg should be treated for high blood pressure even if there are no vascular complications.

It has long been known that kidney disease in diabetes starts with the leaking of certain proteins (albumin) from the blood stream into the urine in increasing quantities. Thereafter, kidney function declines progressively. More recent studies have focused attention on the excretion of very small quantities of albumin (microalbuminuria). Microalbuminuria starts several years before the development of major renal problems. It can also be a warning sign of retinopathy. With special lab tests, we can recognize at an early stage who is at risk of developing these diabetic complications.

Non-Drug Treatment for Hypertensive Diabetics

Lifestyle Changes

Losing excess weight (see Chapter 4) and keeping a healthy lifestyle (see Chapter 5) are essential. They help to decrease blood pressure and improve the control of the blood sugar. Furthermore, the abnormal lipid (fatty substances in the blood) levels common in diabetes can frequently be improved. Decreased salt intake has added benefit because salt retention is a specific problem in diabetes.

Things To Avoid

Certain medications should be avoided. Nonsteroidal anti-inflammatory agents (such as ibuprofen, naproxen or indomethacin) can have an adverse effect on kidney function in diabetes. Corticosteroids (cortisone, prednisone) can lead to hypertension and decrease the control over blood sugar. Oral decongestants in cold remedies have effects similar to noradrenaline, to which diabetics are particularly sensitive. All these medications can increase both blood pressure and blood sugar.

Consumption of alcoholic beverages can also elevate blood pressure. Furthermore, excessive alcohol intake can lead to serious hypoglycemia in diabetics treated with insulin.

Table 13-1: Medications for Treating Hypertension in Patients with Diabetes

First–line medications, in order of preference
ACE inhibitors or calcium antagonists or alpha-blockers
Second–line medications (used with precautions)
Thiazide-like diuretics or beta-blockers
Fall-back medications
Centrally acting agents and vasodilators, when other drugs are contraindicated, cause unacceptable side-effects, or the blood pressure is difficult to control.

Table 13-2: Conditions That Can Be Aggravated by Antihypertensive Drugs

Condition	Drug
Control of blood sugar in Type 2 diabetes	High dose of thiazide diuretics; beta-blockers
Suppression of symptoms and recovery of hypoglycemia	Beta-blockers, mostly nonselective
Increase of lipids	Thiazide diuretics; beta-blockers without intrinsic sympathomimetic activity
Hyperkalemia	ACE inhibitors; potassium-sparing diuretics
Impotence	Diuretics; beta-blockers (mostly nonselective); centrally acting agents
Orthostatic hypotension	Alpha-blockers; centrally acting agents; arterial vasodilators

Drug Treatment for Hypertensive Diabetics

As shown in Table 13-1, several medications can be used to treat hypertension in diabetics. Table 13-2 lists specific problems that diabetics face and the drugs that can make them worse.

ACE Inhibitors (See Chapter 9 for more details)

Several studies have shown that these medications decrease albumin leakage in the urine of diabetics. Some of these studies have also demonstrated that they can slow the deterioration of kidney function. ACE inhibitors don't elevate blood sugar or lipids. They can increase blood potassium, and sometimes make the potassium too high, a condition known as hyper-kalemia, particularly in older people with decreased kidney and adrenal function. Generally speaking, however, ACE inhibitors are an excellent choice for the treatment of hyper-tension for diabetics.

Calcium Antagonists (Chapter 10)
Although these medications may increase blood sugar slightly when first taken, they don't do so with long-term use. They are also an excellent choice in the treatment of high blood pressure for people with diabetes.

Alpha-Blockers (Chapter 8)
These drugs don't affect blood sugar, and furthermore, they have advantageous effects on lipids. They can worsen the ten-dency of some diabetics to have the blood pressure go too low on standing (*orthostatic hypotension*). These medications are a good choice for most diabetics, although they have a limited blood pressure-lowering effect when used alone.

Arterial Vasodilators (Chapter 11)
Because they increase the heart rate and cause fluid to be retained in the body when used alone, these medications are usually given with a beta-blocker and a diuretic. They have no bad effects on blood sugar. They sometimes cause orthostatic hypotension.

Potassium-Sparing Diuretics (Chapter 7)
These medications can be given with other diuretics to avoid the loss of potassium. Given alone, however, they may cause increased levels of blood potassium in diabetics, particularly if there is any kidney impairment. They should not be given with ACE inhibitors, which can also cause potassium to rise.

Thiazide-Type Diuretics (Chapter 7)

These medications can increase blood sugar when administered at high doses. They tend to make control more difficult in diabetics who are not taking insulin. Furthermore, thiazides in high doses can elevate cholesterol and triglycerides (major blood lipids). They may also decrease sexual function, a frequent problem among diabetics. However, these medications, particularly in low doses, are still an acceptable choice for treating hypertension in diabetics and are frequently useful in association with ACE inhibitors.

Indapamide, another diuretic, may not have as severe adverse effects. It can be useful if a diuretic is needed for someone with Type 2 diabetes as it also decreases albumin in urine, similar to ACE inhibitors.

Loop Diuretics (Chapter 7)

The role of these powerful diuretics is mainly to diminish salt and water retention in diabetics with kidney or heart failure. Outside these specific situations, their effects on blood pressure are not very potent.

Beta-Blockers (Chapter 8)

Beta-blockers can cause problems in diabetes. First, beta-blockers (mostly nonselective) decrease the symptoms produced by hypoglycemia, which are due in great part to the effects of adrenaline. Diabetic patients with hypoglycemia will therefore have less increase in heart rate and few or no tremors or anxious feelings and require more time to recover from hypoglycemia. Second, adrenaline produced during hypoglycemia can lead to a severe increase in blood pressure if a person is taking a nonselective beta-blocker

Finally, some beta-blockers increase lipids. This effect is less with beta-blockers that have intrinsic sympathomimetic activity (see Chapter 8).

Nevertheless, for those not prone to hypoglycemia, beta-blockers can be useful, especially those that are more selective such as atenolol, metoprolol and acebutolol.

Centrally Acting Agents (Chapter 8)

These medications do not affect either blood sugar or lipids. Thus, they can be helpful in treating high blood pressure among diabetics. However, they can aggravate orthostatic hypotension and impotence.

Conclusions

Diabetes and hypertension are common companions, and it's important to treat both well. Fortunately, there are good treatments for hypertension that don't interfere with diabetes control; thus, it is usually possible to control both successfully.

WOMEN AND HIGH BLOOD PRESSURE

Douglas R. Ryan, MD, and
Alexander G. Logan, MD

High blood pressure occurs in about 1% of all pregnant women and can cause harm to both the baby and mother. With early diagnosis and treatment, however, we can usually prevent harm. Blood pressure normally falls during pregnancy due to a general relaxing of the mother's blood vessels. It reaches a low point about halfway through the pregnancy and then slowly rises so that at the mother's due date her blood pressure has reached its nonpregnant level. A woman is said to have high blood pressure in pregnancy if her blood pressure

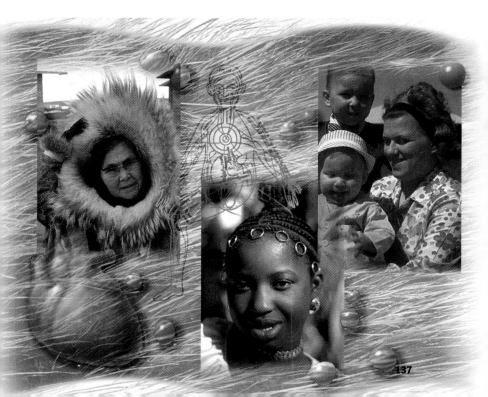

fails to show the usual midpregnancy fall, or if it is consistently greater than 140/90 mm Hg.

Three conditions may produce high blood pressure during pregnancy. The first is chronic high blood pressure, that is, high blood pressure starting before pregnancy. Almost all women of childbearing age with this condition have "essential hypertension", that is, high blood pressure without a cause that can be identified. Women who are hypertensive before they become pregnant can remain hypertensive during their pregnancy. Sometimes their blood pressures may show a steep rise in the last few months of the pregnancy. This poses a danger to mother and fetus alike.

A second condition, called pre-eclampsia, arises only during pregnancy and disappears after the fetus is delivered. Pre-eclampsia is defined as the appearance of high blood pressure, ankle swelling and protein in the urine during the second half of pregnancy. Pre-eclampsia occurs most often in the first pregnancy and uncommonly in subsequent pregnancies. It tends to run in families and occurs more often in mothers with chronic high blood pressure, chronic kidney disease, diabetes, multiple fetuses, and in mothers at the extremes of childbearing age (that is, teenagers or those above 35 years of age). Its exact cause is unknown, but it likely originates in the placenta as a result of a decrease in blood flow to the womb (uterus).

Pre-eclampsia may cause headache, blurred vision and ultimately seizures in the mother. There is often a decrease in the urine production or a build-up in the blood of dietary waste products normally eliminated by the kidneys. Abdominal pain and abnormal blood clotting may occur. In addition the growth of the fetus in the womb may be retarded. Left untreated, severe pre-eclampsia threatens the life of fetus and mother.

The third condition causing high blood pressure during pregnancy is called gestational hypertension. It is defined as high blood pressure without swelling or protein loss in the urine, occurring in a mother who had normal blood pressure before conception. It usually arises in the late stages of pregnancy and resolves within 2 weeks after delivery. It often recurs in later pregnancies.

The term "toxemia" is often used loosely to refer to *any type* of hypertension in pregnancy (most often pre-eclampsia). Since this term is not precisely defined, we recommend that it not be used.

Management of Blood Pressure in Pregnant Women

Regular blood pressure checks are especially important during pregnancy.

When high blood pressure is discovered during pregnancy, your doctor will first determine whether pre-eclampsia is present and, if so, its severity. Women with pre-eclampsia are usually admitted to hospital for observation because this condition can change from mild to severe over 24 to 48 hours. Women with mild pre-eclampsia can be managed with bed rest and drugs that lower elevated pressures. Women with severe pre-eclampsia (severe blood pressure elevation and multiple organs involved) require treatment of their blood pressure with intravenous medication and urgent delivery of the baby as they will not improve until the pregnancy is ended. After delivery most features of pre-eclampsia rapidly disappear, although occasionally they may persist up to 6 months. Fortunately pre-eclampsia does not cause the development of high blood pressure later in life.

Women with gestational high blood pressure are managed in the same manner as those with chronic high blood pressure. Unlike patients with pre-eclampsia, patients with gestational high blood pressure have a higher than average chance of developing high blood pressure later in life. It has been suggested that the tendency to high blood pressure in these women is temporarily unmasked by the stress of pregnancy.

Patients with chronic high blood pressure that becomes worse during pregnancy can often be managed as outpatients. Those who are employed are usually advised to leave their jobs temporarily. All patients are asked to increase the amount of rest they are getting at home. Drugs that lower elevated pressures are then added as necessary. Patients with chronic high blood pressure whose blood pressures are still poorly controlled (diastolic pressure greater than 100) are usually admitted to hospital for bed rest. Delivery is undertaken if the blood pressure is still not controlled or the fetus shows evidence of distress, or, electively, when the fetus is mature. After delivery, higher doses of drugs may be required than before conception.

Treatment of chronic high blood pressure does not prevent the added development of pre-eclampsia and your doctor will be constantly watching for this.

Drug Treatments

Uncontrolled high blood pressure during pregnancy requires treatment. Blood pressure-lowering treatment for all types of high blood pressure in pregnancy provides benefit to the mother and possibly the fetus. Most doctors begin medication that lowers elevated pressures when the mother's diastolic blood pressure is 100 mm Hg or greater. The goal is usually a diastolic pressure of 80 to 90 mm Hg because lower blood pressures may be dangerous for the fetus as they may reduce blood flow to the uterus.

At least five different blood pressure-lowering drugs have been well studied for use in pregnancy and are considered to be effective without endangering the development of the fetus. These are methyldopa, hydralazine, and three beta-blockers, oxprenolol, atenolol, and labetolol (see Chapter 8 for more information). Other acceptable drugs, although less extensively studied in pregnancy, are clonidine, prazosin, and nifedipine.

Generally they are reserved for cases where the best studied drugs are ineffective.

Therapy is usually begun with one drug. A second and then a third drug are added if necessary. If the blood pressure cannot be controlled with three drugs, it is unlikely to come down with the addition of more medication and delivery should be undertaken for the mother's safety.

Two types of drugs are usually avoided during pregnancy. Diuretics may increase the risk of low birth weight infants. Angiotensin-converting enzyme inhibitors, such as captopril and enalapril, may cause growth retardation. Other agents, including minoxidil and calcium antagonists (such as diltiazem and verapamil), are not yet considered suitable for use in human pregnancy because their safety during pregnancy has not been shown.

Initial reports suggesting that pre-eclampsia may be prevented with a low dose of aspirin administered early in pregnancy have not been borne out in more recent, large-scale studies.

Blood Pressure Medications and Breast Feeding

Blood pressure-lowering drugs taken after delivery by a mother who is breast feeding are secreted into breast milk in tiny amounts. The daily dose received by a breast-feeding infant is about one in one hundred parts of that used to lower the mother's blood pressure. Not many scientific studies have examined the effects of breast feeding while taking blood pressure medications. However, infants have routinely and successfully breast fed from mothers taking methyldopa, hydralazine, oxprenolol, atenolol and labetolol. Diuretics are still avoided for treatment of high blood pressure after delivery as these drugs may decrease the amount of milk produced by the mother.

Oral Contraceptives

Oral contraceptives (birth control pills) are the most popular and effective form of temporary birth control. Because nothing else now available works as well, "the pill" will likely remain the most frequently used contraceptive for young women wishing to delay pregnancy. Oral contraceptives are also used to treat acne, excess body hair (hirsutism), menstrual irregularities (dysmenorrhea) and noncancerous lumps in the breast. Oral contraceptives must be used with caution, however, because they sometimes cause important adverse effects, including blood pressure increases.

Before prescribing oral contraceptives, your physician will first enquire about your medical history and present health and discuss the risks and benefits of each method of contraception. Oral contraceptives should not be prescribed to women with a history of thrombophlebitis (the formation of blood clots in the veins), stroke, heart attack, liver disease, known or suspected breast cancer, any estrogen-dependent tumour, abnormal uterine bleeding of unknown cause, or pregnancy or suspected pregnancy. Oral contraceptives also should not be prescribed for women over 35 who smoke because, together, these factors lead to a high risk of cardiovascular disease (Table 14-1). High blood pressure is a major part of this pill-associated risk for cardiovascular disease. Another possible mechanism for the high risk is an increased tendency of the blood to clot. A third mechanism may involve changes in blood fats (lipids) caused by the pill. These lipid effects depend on the type and dosage of the hormones in the oral contraceptive. Estrogens have a favourable effect on blood fats by raising the HDL-cholesterol (good cholesterol) and lowering LDL-cholesterol (bad cholesterol). Progestins, also contained in the pill, have the opposite effect.

Blood pressure rises a little in virtually all women who take estrogen-containing oral contraceptives. This rise usually starts 3 to 9 months after beginning the pill but is not enough to matter for most women. Unfortunately, in about 5% of women over a 5-year period of pill use, the rise is enough to push the pressure beyond the 140/90 level. In a small number of women the rise will be abrupt and will cause severe high blood pressure.

The way in which oral contraceptives cause high blood pressure is unknown. Most women gain weight when put on the pill and salt and water retention in body tissue has been suggested as the cause of their increased blood pressure. The incidence of high blood pressure is lower when "mini-pills" containing lower doses of estrogen are used.

Guidelines for the safe use of oral contraceptives appear in Table 14-2. High blood pressure is not an absolute reason to avoid using oral contraceptives, but other methods of contraception are preferable if you have high blood pressure. If you are unable to use another method, then medication may be prescribed for you to take in addition to the oral contraceptive to lower your blood pressure. This puts your doctor in the awkward position, however, of prescribing one medication that raises your blood pressure and another that lowers it.

Table 14-1: Situations in Which Oral Contraceptives Would Usually Not Be Prescribed

Medical History of
- Thrombophlebitis (clots)
- Liver disease
- Known or suspected breast cancer
- Estrogen-dependent tumour
- Abnormal uterine bleeding of unknown cause
- Pregnancy
- Smokers over the age of 35

Table 14-2: General Guidelines for Safe Use of Oral Contraceptives

In usual circumstances the following precautions should be taken when the pill is used:

- The lowest effective dose of estrogen should be used
- No more than a 6-month supply should be provided at one time
- The blood pressure should be measured every 6 months or whenever the woman feels ill
- If the blood pressure rises, the pill should be stopped if possible and another form of contraception used
- If the blood pressure does not return to normal within 6 months of stopping the pill, additional investigation and treatment are needed

If your blood pressure rises by more than 10 to 20 mm Hg while you are taking an oral contraceptive, it is usually advisable to stop taking the medication and to choose another method of birth control. Your blood pressure should return to normal within 6 months. If your blood pressure does not return to normal during this period, your physician will make further tests for high blood pressure and may prescribe blood pressure-lowering drugs. Such high blood pressure may not necessarily be caused by the oral contraceptives but may simply have developed about the same time.

Hormone Replacement Therapy

An increasing number of women take estrogen to prevent or lessen menopausal symptoms, to prevent osteoporosis (thinning of the bones), and to reduce the risk of heart disease. The way by which female hormones benefit the cardiovascular system is unknown but may involve favourable modifications of the lipids (fats) in the body. Evidence now suggests that the usually prescribed doses of postmenopausal estrogens, alone or in combination with progestin, either have no effect on blood pressure or even reduce it. These positive effects, however, need to be balanced with the risks that hormonal replacement therapy increases, including risks for gallbladder disease and some forms of cancer. In addition, the risks of hormone replacement therapy are increased if a person has very high blood pressure, or smokes, or has had a stroke. Women considering hormone replacement therapy thus have a complicated decision to make, including their personal values and preferences, and their own personal risks for the disorders that hormones can reduce and the risks for the disorders that hormones can increase. While the decision for each woman must be individualized, at least having well-controlled blood pressure is not a strong reason to forgo hormonal replacement therapy.

CHAPTER 15

HOW YOU CAN KEEP YOUR BLOOD PRESSURE UNDER CONTROL

C. Edward Evans, MB, and R. Brian Haynes, MD, PhD

With the treatments that we have today, no one need suffer the complications of high blood pressure. But, many people do suffer from its effects because they don't follow the treatments prescribed by their doctor. This is tragic, because complications can be prevented by close teamwork between a patient and his or her doctor. This chapter gives you information to help you contribute your share of the teamwork.

We'll begin with some tips for self-help:

1. Take all your medication exactly as prescribed. To help with this:
- Take your pills at the time of regular activities you do each day, such as brushing your teeth. We call this tailoring your treatment to fit your daily schedule.
- Set out all your pills for the week on the first day of each week in a special pill organizer.
- If you miss *any* pills, be sure to let your doctor know on your next visit.

2. Refill your prescription *before* it runs out.

3. Make sure that you have a follow-up appointment with your doctor *before* you leave the office.

4. If you must miss an appointment, call your doctor's office to make another appointment as soon as possible.

5. Always keep an up-to-date list of your medication in your wallet.

6. Don't change the amount of your medication or how often you take it without talking to your doctor. You can help any

adjustments in medication by following these suggestions:
- Let your doctor know about any side-effects.
- Keep track of the times during the day or week when you tend to miss or forget your pills.
- Measure your own blood pressure at home or have it taken at work.

7. Be sure to let your doctor know if you have any problems with, or questions about, the care you're receiving. Let your doctor know how you feel about your care and tell him if you're pleased with it or not.

Myths about High Blood Pressure That Can Lead People To Stop Treatment

Before we discuss the reasons for these recommendations, we'd like to expose a few common myths about high blood pressure.

High Blood Pressure Comes and Goes

As stated earlier in this book, once it begins, high blood pressure is almost always a lifelong condition and will continue to cause problems if it's not treated. So, for the great majority of people with high blood pressure it's necessary to continue treatment every day for the rest of their lives. We know from research studies that people who stop taking the treatment prescribed for them often do so because they don't know this important fact.

There are a few exceptions to the above rule. If your blood pressure is very well controlled on medication and stays well controlled for at least a year, your doctor may be able to reduce the amount of medication or even stop it for a period. If you feel that this may be your situation, it's a good idea to bring it to your doctor's attention. But, it's important to know that your blood pressure should be checked even more often after any reduction in medication to make sure that it stays down because, although you may be able to get by on less medication, high blood pressure seldom goes away permanently.

Another way that high blood pressure can "disappear" is if its cause is removed. Unfortunately, as explained in previous chapters, finding a curable cause for a person's high blood pressure is rare.

High Blood Pressure Causes Symptoms That Tell You When You Need To Take Your Medication

Many people think that they can tell when their blood pressure is up from the way they feel. For example, they believe their blood pressure is up when they are feeling nervous, tense, anxious, when they're red in the face, or when they have a headache or nosebleed. These feelings are not good measures of your blood pressure!

At the time high blood pressure is discovered in most people, no symptoms have occurred and little or no permanent damage has been done. Usually the high blood pressure is detected during a routine blood pressure measurement, at a physical examination or when the blood pressure is checked during a visit to the doctor for some other reason. You can't use symptoms of tenseness — or any other feelings — to guide you in taking your prescribed treatment for hypertension. Only a measurement of the blood pressure itself can tell you this, so you should not wait until you think your pressure is up to take medication. In addition, if you take your medication irregularly, you can cause your blood pressure to go on a "roller-coaster ride" that can, at times, be quite dangerous.

Your Doctor Can Tell Whether or Not You Are Taking Your Medication

It is only natural that people try to take as little medication as possible for their high blood pressure (or any other medical condition, for that matter). This can often result in a somewhat dangerous game being played that goes as follows: first, the person cuts back their medication to, say, half the prescribed dose. Then, on the next visit to the doctor, the patient doesn't mention the reduced dose, hoping that the doctor will find that the blood pressure is well controlled anyway. If the blood pressure is elevated, the doctor then often thinks that the medication that she has prescribed isn't strong enough to do the job, and so the prescription is increased. The patient is now in the position where either he will have to confess to lowering the dose or accept the new prescription and try to guess how much of it he should take to keep the blood pressure controlled.

Research has shown that the most likely reason for poor lowering of blood pressure is that a person hasn't taken all the prescribed medication. Many doctors aren't aware that their patients have taken less than the prescribed amount of treatment. The only way your doctor can tell for sure how much medication you have missed is if you tell him. If you've missed any of your pills, for any reason, be sure to let your doctor know this when you visit.

Better still, you can help to keep the amount of medication prescribed to the smallest amount possible by taking all the medication that has been prescribed and bringing to the doctor a list of blood pressure readings taken between visits.

Side-Effects of Blood Pressure Medications Are Worse Than the Disease

All new medications, by government regulation, have to be thoroughly tested before they can be prescribed. Drugs with serious side-effects (that is, those side-effects that threaten your health) are generally weeded out by this procedure. Because high blood pressure is so common, doctors have a lot of experience with blood pressure drugs and can avoid ones with important or common side-effects. As a result, only about one in five people experiences any side-effects from the medications, and most of these are usually just a nuisance rather than being a danger. Side-effects almost always disappear once the drug is stopped, and because there are many drugs for hypertension, the medication can be changed easily if important or even merely annoying side-effects occur.

Nevertheless, like many people, you may feel a bit worse after you start blood pressure medication. This partly could be because you now know that you have a chronic disease and begin to blame it for many of the aches and pains of everyday existence. It also may take some time for your system to adjust to the medication. You may experience some light-headedness upon standing or a bit of drowsiness or lack of energy after starting some blood pressure lowering pills. But these reactions will usually pass with time as your body becomes used to the lower blood pressure and the new medication.

Most people whose blood pressure is well controlled on medication continue their normal lifestyle without any restrictions. On the other hand, some people do experience side-effects from medication and need a change in dose or drug. The only way that your doctor can know whether your reactions mean your medication needs to be changed is if you let her or him know exactly what you have experienced. You can help your doctor find the best treatment for you by keeping track of any important symptoms you feel may be due to your medication. Write them down between visits so you will be able to describe them clearly when you meet with your doctor.

Many people don't want to bother their doctor by complaining about side-effects or admitting missing pills. This concern about the doctor being too busy to bother or wasting his time is not very wise. We know that patients who like their doctor are less likely to let the doctor know about important complaints than those who aren't so devoted to their doctors. Would you fail to notify the garage if the headlights were not working after your car had been serviced? Of course not! So, be sure to have your side-effects attended to, if and when they occur.

Note: If you do experience side-effects that are not severe, don't stop or change your medication without talking to your doctor first. It goes without saying that if you experience severe side-effects, you should contact your doctor immediately.

High Blood Pressure Is Usually Due to Stress

While acute stress can raise your blood pressure, there's no evidence that stress can produce long-lasting high blood pressure that persists once the stress is removed. Nevertheless, if you are under a lot of stress, it is certainly desirable to resolve it if you can.

Many people, however, feel that if you have high blood pressure, you must "take it easy" and avoid all stress or exertion. Not so! If your blood pressure is controlled by medication, then you can lead a perfectly normal existence. You need take no more time off work because of stress or common complaints like colds than if you did not have high blood pressure. You can take on whatever recreation you like, except, perhaps, heavy weight lifting.

High Blood Pressure Is Due to Bad Diet and Bad Habits; Improving Your Lifestyle Is Better Treatment Than Medication

Excess weight, salt and alcohol can raise blood pressure and reducing these can help get the blood pressure down; they've been discussed in previous chapters. Your doctor may prescribe one or more of these methods as a way to lower the amount of medication that you have to take. If this is the case, do your best to follow the recommendation. But it's important that you realize non-drug treatments are often no substitute for drug treatments if your blood pressure is more than mildly elevated.

Your doctor won't be satisfied with your treatment until your blood pressure is well controlled — and neither should you. If your doctor starts you on a non-drug treatment without also putting you on medication, be sure to attend all follow-up visits. If your blood pressure doesn't fall to normal levels in a few weeks, go along with your doctor's suggestion to go on medication. This is not a failure on your part, it doesn't mean that your high blood pressure is unusual, and it isn't necessary to give up the improvements you have been able to make in your lifestyle.

Remember, hypertension is a completely symptomless and painless disorder. If it's caught early in its course, it stays that way as long as it's kept under control.

What You Can Do To Keep Your Blood Pressure under Good Control

On the surface, keeping your blood pressure under control appears to be simple enough: keep all your appointments and take your treatments as they have been prescribed by your doctor. Because you must carry out these tasks for the rest of your life, however, this may be a lot more difficult than you imagine. In fact, without special help, only one person in five does a really good job of following the prescribed treatment for such a long period. The following steps will help you with the lifelong job of keeping your blood pressure under control.

- Clear up any doubts you may have about following the treatment.
- Use special pill containers.
- Tailor your pill-taking so it fits your usual daily activities.
- Avoid running out of pills.
- Keep an up-to-date list of your medications with you at all times.
- Never leave the doctor's office without setting your next appointment.
- Measure your own blood pressure.
- Build a good working relationship with your doctor.

We will discuss these in turn.

Clear Up Any Doubts You May Have about Following the Treatment

You are not likely to follow your prescription closely if you have important doubts about whether or not you really need to follow the treatment. It's important to develop a strongly positive attitude that you are going to get the most out of the treatments your doctor prescribes. Hypertension has serious consequences if it isn't controlled, and you are at definite risk of its complications as long as your blood pressure remains high. The treatments for it are effective if taken as prescribed. Taking them is a nuisance, possibly can be expensive, and not without risks, but for most people the benefits of treatment far outweigh any disadvantages.

Use Special Pill Containers

Many people find it difficult to remember at 10:00 A.M. whether they took the dose of medication that they usually take at 8:00 A.M. One way to overcome this common problem is to buy a pill container with separate compartments for each day of the week. There are many such devices available from your pharmacist (Fig. 15-1). On the first day of each week, fill each compartment of this container with all the pills that you'll need for the week. Then, if you can't recall later in the day whether you took your morning pill, just look in the compartment for the appropriate day and see whether the pill is present or "missing in action".

Another way is to buy a small pill container that will fit easily into your pocket or purse. Fill it up each morning with your pills for the day. Then if you can't remember whether you took your noon pills, just open the container and peek inside.

If you find that you're missing pills more than once a week, try to identify a pattern. Is it the pills you're supposed to take while at work that you're likely to miss? What about the pills you should take last thing at night? Or are the weekends the

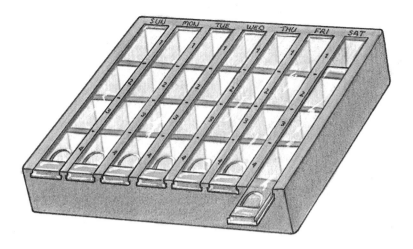

Figure 15-1: Special pill containers can remind you when you've mixed your pills.

most difficult? If you notice a particular time that you're more likely to miss taking your pills, try the following suggestions.

Tailor Your Pill-Taking To Fit into Your Usual Daily Activities
Connect your pill-taking to regular events in your daily schedule so that you take your pills at the same time every day. Do you have any daily habits — something you do every day of the week, whether you go to work or not — such as brushing your teeth every morning? Do you always have a cup of coffee or juice when you get up? Whatever your daily routine might be, link your pill-taking to that event. And, if you must take your pills more than once a day, think of a habit that coincides with those and take your medicine then.

Many people believe that different types of medications need to be taken at completely separate times. In fact, this is seldom so. For example, suppose you are prescribed three different medicines for your high blood pressure, all of which are to be taken once a day. You can (and should) take all of these pills at the same time, unless your doctor or pharmacist advises otherwise. Another good idea is to try to schedule taking your pills when you're more likely to be at home. It's much harder to remember to take pills when away from home because of preoccupation with other activities or embarrassment about taking pills in public places.

If you do have to take your pills while at work, one suggestion already mentioned is to buy a small pill container from your pharmacist that you can keep in your pocket. Another is to keep a small extra supply of pills in your car or at work so you'll always have some on hand if you forget to bring some from home that day.

If you happen to miss a dose and you recall having missed it within a few hours, take it right away unless the next dose is scheduled to follow in a short while.

Never Run Out of Pills

Avoid running out of pills. Sometimes it happens that your doctor doesn't prescribe enough to last you until the next appointment, or you may have to postpone an appointment and your pills run out before the rescheduled time. You may even feel that it won't make much difference if you stop the pills for a few days — after all, shouldn't your body take a rest from the pills occasionally? While this may sound logical, it's incorrect and potentially dangerous. In the first place, your body needs the medicine to keep your blood pressure under control. Second, in some instances, stopping the medication suddenly can lead to sharp, severe rises in blood pressure that can be harmful. It isn't wise to stop your medication without your doctor's recommendation and careful measurement of your blood pressure. Therefore, if you ever find yourself without enough pills to last until your next appointment, make sure to have your prescription filled before it runs out.

Here are some ways to avoid running out:

• When you visit your doctor, don't leave without a prescription for enough medication to last at least until your next scheduled visit.

• When you are about to go on a vacation or trip, remember to take along all the medication you'll need, with a good margin for an unexpected delay. Make sure you pack your pills someplace where you can easily get them at the right time.

• If you are about to run out of pills, either call your pharmacist and ask him to call your doctor for a renewal or call your doctor's office directly, leaving the exact details of your prescription plus the phone number of the pharmacy. In either case, it is wise to allow 2 or 3 days for the prescription to be renewed. But, if you do happen to run out before you notice it and you are unable to reach your doctor, your pharmacist will often provide you with enough pills to last you until the doctor can be contacted.

Keep an Up-to-Date List of Your Medications with You at All Times

It's a good idea to keep an up-to-date record of your medications in your wallet or purse. There are several good reasons for this. Knowing something about the medications that you take can help make you feel more in control. If you're in an accident or become ill and require emergency medical aid, this information could be of vital importance in your care. Should you lose or misplace your medication, especially if you're away from home, having a list handy can turn a possible disaster into a minor inconvenience. If you change doctors for any reason or are referred to another doctor for care of any problem, including your high blood pressure, your new doctor will want to know exactly what medications you have been prescribed. You also can use your list to check the accuracy of the prescription label when your medications are renewed.

To make it easier to follow this advice, ask your doctor or pharmacist to write down your medications on a piece of paper or a card. Or, write them down yourself by copying them from the pill bottles you're given by the pharmacist. If you do this, ask your doctor or pharmacist to check your list. Of course, you should revise this list every time the medications are changed. It's a good idea to put the list in a medical alert pendant.

Never Leave the Doctor's Office without Setting Up Your Next Appointment

It's important never to leave your doctor's office without a specific appointment for your next visit, and, if at all possible, never miss an appointment. It's easy to drop out of care, and this is the most common cause of people failing to get and keep their blood pressure under control. If you don't have a specific appointment time and date when you leave your doctor's office, there's a good chance that you'll forget to make a new appointment at the appropriate time later.

With the active and busy lives most of us lead, remembering appointments can be a real problem. This is even more difficult if the date is several weeks or months in advance. If your doctor's office doesn't have an automatic reminder system (and most don't), then try developing one yourself. Each time you visit your doctor, be sure to write down the details of your next appointment before you leave. Even if the receptionist offers you the "opportunity" of calling back later for the next appointment, ask for a specific date and time if at all possible. If this isn't possible, write a reminder to yourself in your calendar or post it on the refrigerator. List the month and day, not "in 2 month's time", as you can easily forget which 2 months. When you get closer to the appointed time, then you can call to confirm it.

By the way, if you do miss an appointment, it's unlikely that the doctor's office staff will contact you. Most doctors consider it your responsibility to re-book missed appointments.

Keep Track of Your Blood Pressure

Many people find it helpful to see how well they're keeping their blood pressure under control. This provides feedback that can help to motivate your efforts to follow the treatment prescribed and may help with adjustments of your treatment.

Aside from the blood pressures taken when you visit your doctor's office, you can get more pressures taken at work if you're employed at a place with a nurse or other medical staff on duty. Many doctors also allow (and encourage) you to drop into the clinic for a quick blood pressure check by the clinic nurse. Keep a record of all these blood pressures and show them to your doctor at your next visit. Aside from the picture they give you of your blood pressure control, they can provide your doctor with valuable information for adjusting your medications. This is because blood pressure varies a great deal from time to time, and readings taken outside the doctor's office are often a more accurate reflection of true blood pressure. The larger the number of blood pressure readings available to your doctor when decisions are made, the easier it will be to decide.

Measure Your Own Blood Pressure

For many people with hypertension, there are good reasons to invest in equipment to take your own blood pressure at home. The Canadian Coalition for High Blood Pressure Prevention and Control recommends self-measurement of blood pressure, under the guidance of a health care provider, in the following patients:

• Those who show labile (changing) or elevated blood pressure in the health care provider's office;
• Those with poorly controlled hypertension;
• Those who wish to play a greater role in their own care;
• Those who require an assessment of their antihypertensive therapy (blood pressure medication) because of concerns about excessive blood pressure lowering or insufficient duration of drug action.

Some people have high blood pressure time and again in the doctor's office, but when their blood pressure is measured away from the clinic, at home or at work, it's normal. We now know this "white coat" or "office" hypertension may not be as harmful as blood pressure that is high all the time. Home blood pressure measurement may be helpful in sorting out whether you have this type of high blood pressure, although the exact role of home blood pressure readings in care has not been clearly shown.

If your doctor has suggested you take your pressure at home, or you would like to do it for your own interest, the first questions usually are: which blood pressure machine should I get? and where should I get it? One type of instrument has a column of mercury and is known technically as a *mercury sphygmomanometer* (Fig. 15-2). Most people will recog-

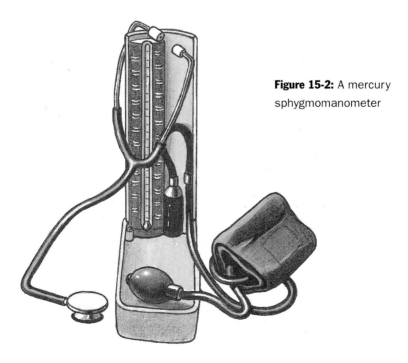

Figure 15-2: A mercury sphygmomanometer

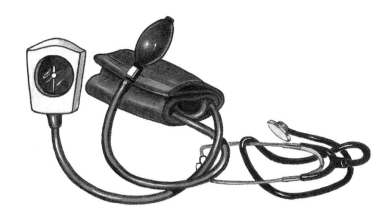

Figure 15-3: An aneroid sphygmomanometer

nize this as the type most commonly used by health professionals. The next most common type is the *aneroid sphygmomanometer*, which usually has a small round dial instead of a mercury column (Fig. 15-3). You need a stethoscope to use either of these machines.

As well there are many machines sold specially for home measurement. Many have digital displays: most don't require the use of a stethoscope. Some automatically blow up the cuff and even deflate it. Some print out the pulse rate, systolic and diastolic blood pressures, date and time, and even have a built-in alarm clock!

The most reliable and accurate type of machine, when it's used properly, is the mercury sphygmomanometer. This type is used as the standard against which other devices are measured. The main drawbacks with mercury devices are that they are cumbersome and quite heavy, the mercury can spill out if the device is turned upside down or broken and mercury can be toxic (never use a vacuum cleaner to pick up spilt mercury, it vaporizes the mercury). Added to this is the fact that you need to use a stethoscope, place it correctly on the arm, and listen for the sounds in the artery while reading the gauge and simultaneously deflating a cuff wrapped around one of your arms. Although this is the standard method of measuring blood pressure, most people will find one of the other methods described below more convenient and just as useful.

A good quality aneroid device is probably the most economic method of measuring blood pressure. The advantage of an aneroid instrument over the mercury one is that it's much smaller and easier to handle and doesn't have the potential problem of mercury toxicity. It still requires the use of a stethoscope and juggling with deflation valves while reading the circular gauge. These instruments can become inaccurate with rough usage, but you may be able to take it back to your supplier or doctor and have it calibrated against (yes, you guessed it) a mercury sphygmomanometer. It should be checked at least twice a year.

With both the mercury and aneroid machines you need practice at measuring blood pressure the correct way. Table 15-1 outlines the approved method of taking blood pressure, but you will most likely need someone who is familiar with taking blood pressure to show you how to do it. Don't give up if you find it difficult at first, most doctors and nurses couldn't hear a thing either when they were first taught to take blood pressures!

What about all the other fancy machines you see for sale (such as the one in Fig.15-4) in department store catalogues, drugstores, electronic stores, and even advertised with your gas credit card bill? They certainly look attractive, hi-tech and simple to use, and usually don't need a stethoscope. If they are as accurate as the digital readout display leads you to believe, they could be the no-fuss answer, especially for people with hearing problems. Buyer beware! Some of these machines are so inaccurate that they can be positively dangerous. But there are so many potential advantages to an easy-to-use, automatic machine that we can't dismiss them out of hand. If you do get one, be sure to have its accuracy checked against a mercury device when you first get it and have it checked regularly thereafter.

About 10 years ago we carried out a detailed study of

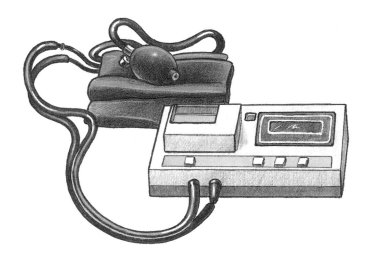

Figure 15-4: An electronic home blood pressure device

home blood pressure machines, which was published in the *Journal of Hypertension* (February 1989). We tested 23 different devices and found *only seven* that we judged suitable for home use. More recently, in May 1992, the Consumers' Union of the United States published a review of home blood pressure monitors in their magazine, *Consumer Reports*. They listed 18 devices that appear to be reasonably accurate, ranging in price from $20 U.S. to $130 U.S. It is important to note that machines that measure blood pressure on an index finger are so unreliable that they are unacceptable. This article should be available in your local public library and is well worth reading before you take the plunge.

Other points worth noting:

• Machines using microphones as the listening device have to be more carefully positioned on the arm than those using an oscillometer (a second bladder inside the cuff).
• Any machine for self-measurement of blood pressure should have a cuff that's specially made to be applied with one hand. Most use a bar called a D-ring and Velcro® fasteners to make application easier.

- Electronic machines can give erratic readings when the batteries are getting low, and this usually happens *before* the battery indicator lets you know that the batteries need changing.
- Even though a good set of instructions may come with the machine, it's important to review how to use it with someone who is well versed in taking blood pressures, such as your doctor or nurse.
- It's important to make sure you have the correct cuff size for your arm (see Table 15-1).
- Most electronic instruments are delicate, and if you drop one you should have its accuracy checked.
- Automatic blood pressure machines have real difficulty getting accurate readings if you have an irregular pulse or if your pulse is very slow.
- If you buy any blood pressure machine, insist on the right to return it if you're unable to get good readings at home or if it appears to be inaccurate when tested against your doctor's blood pressure machine.

If you do collect blood pressure readings between visits to your doctor, be sure to record the date and time of day, and show the results to your doctor. You can write down the pressure in a pocket calendar, along with any pills you may have missed and any side-effects you feel may have been due to the medication. This will make it possible to cover all these matters quickly with your doctor.

Blood pressure varies quite a bit from day to day and even from one hour to the next. For example, your blood pressure may be 140/96 on one reading and 120/80 the next. It's quite usual for the lower number of each of these two readings (that is, 96 and 80, the diastolic blood pressures) to vary within a range of 20 — say, from 80 to 100 or 70 to 90. Because of this change from one time to the next, blood pressure is always taken as the average of several readings over a period of days or weeks. This is one of the reasons why it can be valuable for

Table 15-1: How to Measure Blood Pressure

1. If you are using a mercury sphygmomanometer, the top of the column should be at eye level. With an aneroid sphygmomanometer, the indicator should start at zero or very close to it.

2. Use a cuff that is the right size, measured around the mid-upper arm:

Adult arm size	Bladder size
less than 33 cm (13 inches)	12 x 23 cm (5 x 9 inches)
33 - 41 cm (13 - 16 inches)	15 x 33 cm (6 x 13 inches)
more than 41 cm (16 inches)	18 x 36 cm (7 x 14 inches)

3. Place the cuff with the lower edge 3 cm above the crease of your elbow with the bladder centred just inside your biceps muscle. You should be comfortable, with your arm bared and well supported.

4. Don't talk or cross your legs during measurement; these can raise blood pressure readings.

5. Place the head of the stethoscope gently but firmly over the inside of your biceps muscle, just below the cuff. (If you squeeze this area with your fingers, you should be able to feel the brachial artery pulsating just to the body side of your biceps muscle, a little above the crease of your elbow.)

6. Raise the pressure in the cuff about 30 mm Hg above your usual systolic pressure.

7. Open the valve to let the air out slowly, about 2 mm per heart beat.

8. Record the systolic pressure (the first appearance of a clear tapping sound) and diastolic pressure (the point at which the tapping sound disappears) (Fig.15-5).

9. Ignore any isolated extra heart beats or noises other than the regular tapping heart sounds.

10. Leaving the cuff partially inflated for too long may make the sounds disappear due to venous congestion. To avoid this, at least 30 seconds should elapse between readings. If the sounds are faint, raise your arm, milk down the forearm (i.e., encircle it with your fingers and firmly stroke down), and, with your arm still raised, inflate the cuff. Lower your arm and proceed to take your pressure.

11. If there is consistently higher pressure in one arm than the other, use the arm with the higher pressure.

your doctor to have you record blood pressures between office visits. If these readings are accurate, they will provide more information on which to judge your average blood pressure.

It's important for you to know that this variability in blood pressure exists so you don't become concerned about it or react incorrectly to it. Don't try to change your medication on the basis of the readings that you get, and don't be surprised if your blood pressure is up when you feel well or down when you feel tense. Rely on your doctor to interpret your blood pressures and you can be sure your readings will help make his job easier.

If you're monitoring your own blood pressure, you should discuss with your doctor how low a pressure he feels you should aim for. For most people, the goal is to keep the average diastolic blood pressure below 90 and the systolic pressure below 140.

Build an Effective Working Relationship with Your Doctor

Since you can expect that you'll require lifelong care for your hypertension, it's important to establish a good relationship with your doctor. As with all relationships, this will require a mutual effort if it's to be fully successful.

Most patients look for a doctor with whom they can talk and who is interested in listening to their concerns. You should not be afraid to ask questions about your condition. Most doctors will respond positively when they realize that you have genuine questions and concerns. For example, if you've been following a prescribed treatment faithfully and your blood pressure remains persistently elevated, it's important to ask your doctor whether there is something more that can be done (including a referral to a specialist).

It's important to be honest and open with your doctor and to build a working relationship that will allow you to achieve all the benefits of modern therapy. This could be the beginning

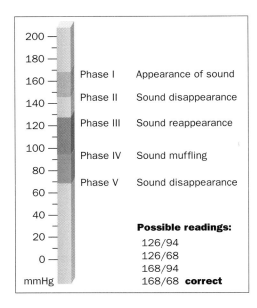

200 —		
180 —		
160 —	Phase I	Appearance of sound
140 —	Phase II	Sound disappearance
120 —	Phase III	Sound reappearance
100 —	Phase IV	Sound muffling
80 —		
60 —	Phase V	Sound disappearance
40 —		
20 —		**Possible readings:**
0 —		126/94
mmHg		126/68
		168/94
		168/68 **correct**

Figure 15-5:
Korotkoff phases

of a long and rewarding association. As in all relationships, if you're pleased with the care you're receiving, let your doctor know —you'll make his or her day. But, if you find you can't relate to your doctor and aren't getting the interest in or answers to your questions, get another doctor. After all, everyone has a different personality, and sometimes it takes a while to get a good match.

Bibliography
Blood pressure monitors. *Consumer Reports*, (May 1992):295–9.

Canadian Coalition for High Blood Pressure Prevention and Control. Recommendations on self-measurement of blood pressure. *Canadian Medical Association Journal*, Vol. 138, No. 12 (15 June 1988):1093–6.

Evans CE, Haynes RB, Goldsmith CH, Hewson SA. Home blood pressure measuring devices: a comparative study of accuracy. *Journal of Hypertension*, Vol. 7 (1989):133–42.